A Color

MW00723545

Gastroenterology

A Color Handbook of

Gastroenterology

HJF Hodgson
Claire Cousins
Hammersmith Hospital and
Imperial College School of Medicine
London, UK

Ralph Boulton
North Middlesex Hospital
London, UK

Sanjeev Gupta
Albert Einstein College of Medicine
Yeshiva University
Bronx NY, USA

McGraw-Hill
Health Professions Division

New York   St. Louis   San Francisco   Auckland   Bogotá
Caracas   Lisbon   London   Madrid   Mexico City
Milan   Montreal   New Delhi   San Juan   Singapore
Sydney   Tokyo   Toronto

McGraw-Hill

A Division of The **McGraw·Hill** *Companies*

Published in the United States of America in 2000 by
The McGraw-Hill Companies, Inc.,
1221 Avenue of the Americas,
New York, NY 10020

ISBN: 0–8385–1623–8

Library of Congress Cataloging in Publication Data is available for this title

Copyright © 2000 Manson Publishing Ltd.,
73 Corringham Road,
London NW11 7DL, UK

Project management: John Ormiston
Colour reproduction: Jade Reprographics, Braintree, England
Printed by: Grafos SA, Barcelona, Spain

The pictures shown on the front cover are, from top left: **50**, normal histology of stomach; **78**, lymphoma of
stomach; **64**, gastric cancer; **69**, ingested foreign body; **86**, histology of normal villi; **153**, systemic vasculitis; **92**, chronic zinc deficiency; **168**, neuroendocrine tumor of the liver; **236**, pseudomembranous colitis.
On the back cover, from top left: **131**, completed spout ileostomy; **24**, nut-cracker esophagus; **207**, polyps.

Contents

Contents

Preface

The practice of gastroenterology requires perhaps the broadest mix of skills of any of the many subspecialties of internal medicine. The range of symptomatology, the involvement of a variety of abdominal organs, the spectrum of disease processes and the diversity of investigative techniques provide both the challenge and excitement of the subject.

Clearly, the format of this book reflects the major importance of the visual aspects of the subject, both for diagnosis and for understanding. Modern gastroenterologists have at their finger tips the powerful investigative tool of endoscopy, and in collaboration with colleagues in the imaging departments, have the ability to recognise abnormality or confirm normality in most intestinal and abdominal organs. However, the practice of gastroenterology extends far beyond that; we hope this book equally explains and emphasises the nature of the disease processes, the aetiology, the epidemiology, pathology, and pathophysiology of gastrointestinal diseases and perhaps above all the approach to the patient.

This book is aimed at trainees. We hope that it will help both those who wish to make gastroenterology their subspecialty, and those who wish to hold gastroenterology as one component of their internal medicine expertise. We hope that residents and clinical fellows, senior house officer and specialist registrars will find it as useful as we hope we have made it. Clearly, a short book of this nature cannot cover all the small print. Nonetheless, we hope the principles are sufficiently clear to provide a firm basis for future study and wider experience.

Acknowledgements

We are grateful to a number of our colleagues for providing illustrative material, either by providing material from their own collection, or because their expertise allowed the procedures to be performed in the first instance. These include Dr James Jackson, Professor John Calam, Dr Julian Walters, Dr Simon Taylor-Robinson, Mr John Spencer, Mr Witold Kmiot, Dr AJW Hilson, Dr Shirley Hodgson, Mr Mohammed Aslam, Dr Simon Olliff, Dr N de Souza, Professor Michael Peters.

We would also like to thank Dr Roy Cockel, Selly Oak Hospital, University Hospital Trust, Birmingham, UK, for allowing us to publish some of his endoscopic images.

Major Presenting Complaints

from the caecum is plum-coloured or darker. Low-grade chronic blood loss may be invisible (occult) and present with anaemia.

ABNORMAL BOWEL HABIT

Normal bowel habit varies between people, from two or three loose stools daily to hard motions every second or third day. Changes in pre-existing pattern are more significant than long-standing deviation from what the patient or doctor considers 'normal'.

Constipation

This is described as infrequent passage of stools which become dehydrated and hard from a long stay in the colon. Trivial causes include immobility, diminished food intake, and medication with constipating agents, e.g. codeine. Constipation associated with epigastric pain may be due to ingestion of calcium or aluminium-containing antacids. Constipation requires further investigation when recent in origin or associated with colicky pain. Absolute constipation followed by distension is a cardinal feature of intestinal obstruction. Hypercalcaemia and myxoedema can present with constipation.

Diarrhoea

This requires careful definition. Diarrhoea may describe states from moderate to frequent passage of formed stools to massive volumes of liquid stool. Many patients with a 'diarrhoeal' form of irritable bowel have two to three loose motions in the morning, usually after food, but the total mass of stool is normal. Diarrhoea waking a patient at night is generally significant. Passage of blood and mucus is obviously significant, but passage of mucus alone does not indicate pathology. Clinical indications of steatorrhoea (pale, floating, foul-smelling) (see 8) are unreliable indicators of excess fat (malabsorption). Observation of rainbow colours on the surface of the stool or lavatory pan water implies severe steatorrhoea – such as seen in pancreatic insufficiency or extensive small gut resection. Inflammatory colitis, or ischaemic change in the colon, is often associated with crampy abdominal colic, but disease of the small intestine can also cause colonic colic as excess fluid enters the colon.

Under normal circumstances, less than 1.25 l of intestinal fluid leaves the ileum to enter the colon, which then reduces the volume to less than 300 ml. Liquid stool volumes of over 1.5 l a day therefore strongly suggest disease of the small gut.

RECTAL SYMPTOMS

Symptoms from the rectum include:
- Tenesmus: this refers to a feeling of rectal fullness and a sensation that the bowel needs evacuation (even if a bowel motion has recently been passed). It reflects the presence of rectal inflammation.
- Constant anal pain (suggesting the presence of an abscess or thrombosed haemorrhoid).
- A tearing pain on defaecation (suggesting an anal fissure).
- Proctalgia fugax: an intense intermittent anal pain attributed to spasm.
- Pruritus ani: anal itch, which occurs idiopathically or in the presence of pinworm infection.

WEIGHT LOSS

In combination with other gastrointestinal symptoms, this is a major symptom. Systemic conditions (thyrotoxicosis, tuberculosis, diabetes, cancer and anxiety) should also be considered.

OTHER GASTROINTESTINAL SYMPTOMS

Other less well-defined complaints should be considered. Abdominal distension, particularly after meals, is one classical manifestation of functional bowel disease, probably reflecting delayed emptying of small intestinal contents into the caecum. Other irritable bowel syndrome manifestations include alternation between constipation and diarrhoea, colicky colonic pain, intermittent discomfort in the right upper quadrant, left upper quadrant or left lower quadrant of the abdomen. Long-standing symptoms in the presence of otherwise good health, dating back many years, or an acute attack of gastroenteritis following which persistent abnormality of bowel habit persists, are suggestive clinical features for diagnosis of irritable bowel.

Physical Examination

Table 1. General physical signs of gastrointestinal disease	
Hands	
Liver palms	Acute or chronic liver disease
Clubbing (**1,2**)	Cirrhosis, Crohn's disease
Leukonychia (white nails)	Liver disease, protein-losing enteropathy
Dupuytren's contracture	Alcoholism
Skin	
Spider naevi	Cirrhosis or hepatitis
White spots	Chronic liver disease (**3**)
Pigmentation (**3**)	Haemochromatosis, internal malignancy, malabsorption
Blisters, depigmentation	Porphyria cutanea tarda
Erythema nodosum (**4**)	Inflammatory bowel disease
Eyes	
Coloration	Jaundice (**5**)
Episcleritis (**6**)/iritis	Inflammatory bowel disease (**2**)
Retinal appearances	Pseudoxanthoma elasticum
Venous pressure	Hepatic pain in congestive cardiac failure
	Cardiological causes of ascites or protein-losing enteropathy
Lymphadenopathy	Carcinoma of the stomach and other malignancies
Cyanosis	Severe liver disease
Anaemia	Acute and chronic gastrointestinal blood loss
Cardiac disease and peripheral pulses	Intestinal angina, ischaemic gut disease, mesenteric emboli
Gynaecomastia	Chronic liver disease
Peripheral neuropathy	Alcoholism, amyloidosis, porphyria, B_{12} deficiency due to malabsorption
Encephalopathy	Liver disease
Erythema *ab igne* (7) (mottled pigmentation of the skin due to application of external heat)	Chronic pain

The historical features outlined above will have suggested a short differential diagnosis, and in many patients with gastrointestinal disease no abnormal physical findings will be demonstrable. Nonetheless, a physical examination, which should not be confined only to the abdomen, should be made. Aspects of the general physical examination that may provide useful clues to gastroenterological and hepatic conditions are given in *Table 1* (**1–7**).

Physical Examination

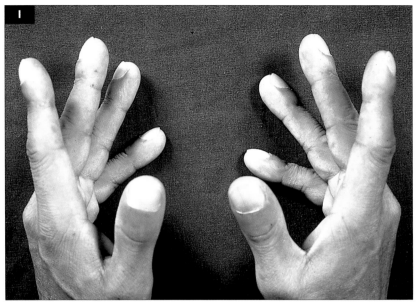

1 Clubbing of the fingers.

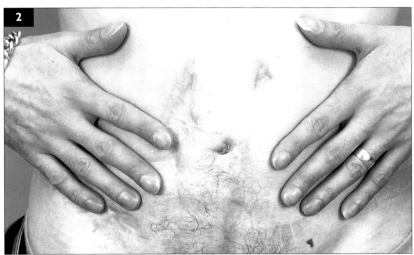

2 Clubbing and multiple scars point to chronic inflammatory bowel disease.

Physical Examination

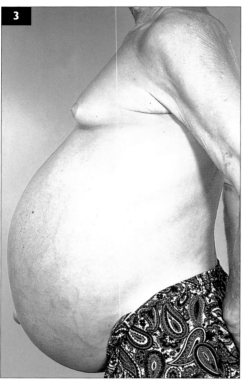

3 Gynaecomastia, ascites and pigmentation all point to chronic liver disease in this patient.

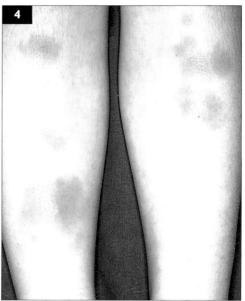

4 Erythema nodosum, seen in Crohn's disease or ulcerative colitis.

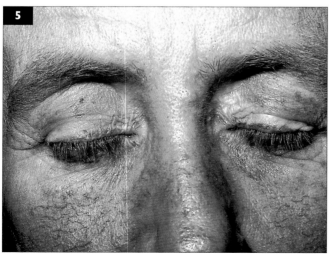

5 Jaundice; xanthelasma around the eyes in chronic cholestatic jaundice (primary biliary cirrhosis).

Physical Examination

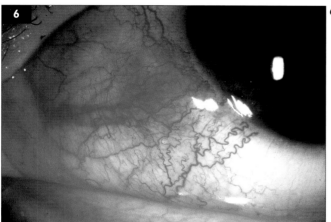

6 Episcleritis, another association of active inflammatory bowel disease.

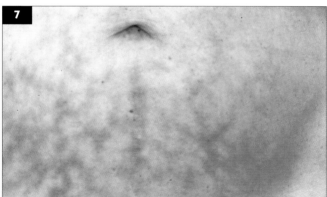

7 Erythema *ab igne*, due to applied heat in an attempt to relieve chronic pain in a patient with a narrow terminal ileum causing recurrent abdominal pain.

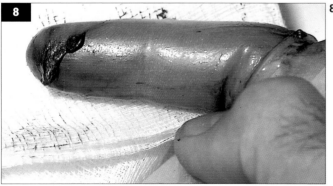

8 'Silver stool' – the pale steatorrhoeic stool, together with the presence of altered blood, in a patient with a combination of obstructive jaundice and bleeding into the gut.

Physical Examination

LIVER

An enlarged, tender liver may be inflamed, congested or the site of an abscess or tumour. The patency of the hepatic venous drainage can be checked by showing elevation of the jugular venous pressure on pressing over the liver. Although a crude physical sign, there is a good correlation between the finding of a fibrous, hard liver and cirrhosis. Rapid changes in liver size may indicate mobilisation of fat, and in alcoholic patients the liver may diminish in size rapidly on abstention from alcohol. A hepatic bruit may be heard in alcoholic hepatitis or in patients with tumours.

SPLEEN

Palpating the spleen can be difficult: rotating the patient on to the right side, with a helping examiner's hand in the left flank, and deep inspiration may all help the examining fingers.

ASCITES

While gross ascites is easy to detect (3), one may be misled into diagnosing ascites in gross obesity, as fat is liquid at room temperature. Minor degrees of ascites can be difficult to detect clinically, but ultrasound examination will settle any doubt.

ABDOMINAL BRUITS

Bruits in the epigastrium are not necessarily pathological, as the superior mesenteric artery may often be stretched over the pancreas. Nonetheless, they should lead to consideration of a diagnosis of intestinal ischaemia or a pancreatic tumour.

HERNIAL ORIFICES, SCARS

Hernial orifices and scars are relevant in the context of colicky abdominal pain, as they may indicate obstruction in the hernial sac or due to adhesions.

Chapter Two

Mouth and Pharynx

Examining the mouth may show signs suggestive of gastrointestinal disease

The appearances of the tongue can reflect vitamin deficiencies

Mouth ulcers may reflect coeliac disease or Crohn's disease

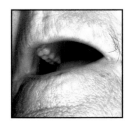 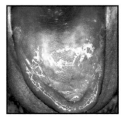 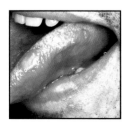 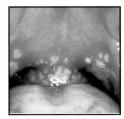

Oral Problems

The mouth is the most easily examined part of the gastrointestinal tract. Important clues to systemic illness and to disease elsewhere in the gut can be manifest in the mouth.

CHEILITIS/ANGULAR STOMATITIS
Inflammation of the corner of the mouth (9) can be due to a number of causes. Chronic candidal infection is frequent in endentulous patients; streptococcal and staphylococcal infections are more common in those with teeth. Riboflavin deficiency (vitamin B_2) causes a smooth 'magenta' tongue and angular stomatitis and, eventually, paraesthesia, photophobia and blurred vision.

GEOGRAPHIC TONGUE
An oval or 'map'-shaped area on the dorsum of the tongue with a well-defined margin and no known cause. Asymptomatic, but some patients complain of sensitivity to spicy foods. Patients should be reassured.

GLOSSITIS
A red painful tongue can be caused by candida infection and by deficiency of iron, B_{12}, folate or riboflavin ('magenta tongue') (10).

APHTHOUS ULCERS
Mouth ulcers (11) can be intensely painful lesions.

Epidemiology and aetiology
About 20% of the population suffer mouth ulcers, and the point prevalence is 2%. Most present in the first two decades of life. Females are slightly more frequently affected than males. One-third of patients recognise foods as triggering attacks. Cessation of smoking may also provoke episodes.

Special forms Minor aphthae: the most common form, appearing every couple of months in crops. Lesions are 1–10 mm and round or ovoid with a 'punched-out' appearance, and only affect the gingival and hard palate – the non-keratinised epithelium. The lesions heal after 3–14 days, usually without scarring.

Major aphthae: lesions are larger than minor aphthae and can last longer – up to several months, sometimes scarring.

Herpetiform aphthae: named after the resemblance to herpetic lesions, crops of up to 100 small 2–3-mm lesions are scattered throughout the mouth.

Differential diagnosis
A number of gastrointestinal diseases can manifest as recurrent oral ulceration. These include Crohn's disease, coeliac disease, Behçet's disease, and, less floridly, ulcerative colitis.

Laboratory and special examinations
Deficiency of iron, folate and vitamin B_{12} must be excluded.

Pathophysiology
The cause is unknown. There is speculation regarding viral initiation, or an autoimmune reaction based on cross-reactivity between food and bacterial antigens. A weak association with HLA-A2 is reported. The inflammatory infiltrate is lymphocytic and monocytic.

Prognosis
Crops of minor aphthae can recur for years, major aphthae may be more frequent and persist for longer. Episodes of herpetiform aphthae desist after a few years.

Management options
Acute episodes are treated with tetracycline mouthwashes, topical anaesthetic lozenges, and topical anti-inflammatory agents to relieve the pain. Corticosteroids can be given as pastes or pellets or rarely systemically for severe disease.

Nutritional deficiency should be sought and corrected. Progesterone may benefit the minority of women with menstrual-related symptoms.

Oral Problems

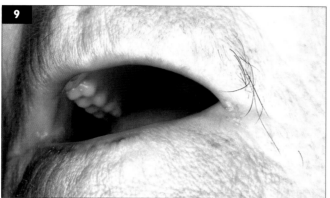

9 Cheilitis; painful areas at the corner of the mouth, in a patient with chronic iron deficiency.

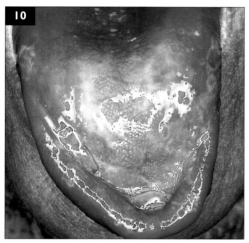

10 A smooth, painful tongue of vitamin B deficiency.

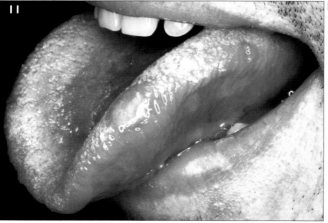

11 Aphthous ulcer – suggesting inflammation in the bowel (Crohn's disease, coeliac disease).

Oral Cancer

History
Patients complain of an enlarging lump or ulcer. Lesions may bleed and are initially painless.

Physical examination
Exophytic and ulcerating lesions are seen. Although these lesions can arise anywhere in the mouth and pharynx, 50% involve the lips or tongue. Multiple lesions are not uncommon.

Epidemiology and aetiology
The disease is more common in men than in woman, and the average age at presentation is 60 years. The major factors in causation are smoking and chewing tobacco, and drinking alcohol. Other factors are chronic irritation from ill-fitting dentures, and chronic infections such as candida and syphilis (**12**). Leukoplakia and, in the Far East, submucous fibrosis (associated with chewing tobacco, betel and eating chilies) are premalignant conditions.

Differential diagnosis
Other causes of oral ulceration. There are no specific features, so all oral ulcers of more than 2 weeks' duration must be biopsied. An indurated ulcer base and hard everted edges are suggestive of carcinoma.

Laboratory and special examinations
Histological assessment is mandatory.

Pathophysiology
About 90% of lesions are squamous cell carcinomas that spread by local invasion. Distant metastases are rare.

Prognosis
Poor.

Management options
Alcohol and tobacco must be discontinued, as there is a 20% chance of a second head and neck cancer. En-bloc resection and radiotherapy offer the best chance of prolonged survival.

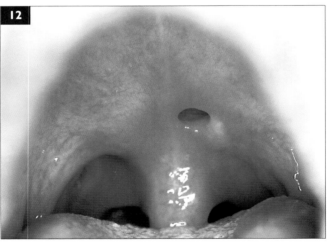

12 A perforated hard palate – the Gumma of tertiary syphilis.

Oral Keratoses and Leukoplakia

KERATOSES
Excessive keratinisation of the oral mucosa presents as a white patch. It occurs in a number of conditions including:
- Chronic irritation (smoking, poorly fitting dentures).
- Idiopathic leukoplakia.
- Lichen planus.
- Lupus erythematosus.
- Candidal infection.
- Hairy leukoplakia.

If white lesions cannot be scraped off (as for instance with candidal pseudomembranes) and other causes are excluded, it is termed leukoplakia.

LEUKOPLAKIA
This is a premalignant lesion; up to 5% progress to cancer – especially lesions on the floor of the mouth and those with erythema. Biopsy is mandatory, thermal surgery and topical cytotoxic therapy are management options.

LICHEN PLANUS
A benign lesion, the most common intraoral keratosis, which can manifest anywhere in the mouth and tongue.

History
Oral lesions are usually asymptomatic and found incidentally, often during dental examination (in contrast to skin lesions that are pruritic).

Physical examination
Reticular or papular lesions. Wickham's striae – a reticulated fine lacy white pattern over the lesions – are characteristic. Concurrent cutaneous lesions are violaceous, with a polygonal planar lesion found particularly on the flexor aspect of the wrists and ankles.

Epidemiology and aetiology
After the third decade.

Special forms
- Hypertrophic: often asymptomatic.
- Erosive: large shallow painful ulcers that can be complicated by infection.
- Bullous: rare. If bullae burst they form ulcers.

Differential diagnosis
Local lichenified eruptions are associated with drugs, and some dental amalgams. Leukoplakia, erythroplakia.

Laboratory and special examinations
Histology shows hyperkeratosis, hyperplasia, and liquefaction of the basal cell layer. Dense lymphocytic infiltration of the dermoepidermal junction.

Pathophysiology
Unknown. It may be precipitated by drugs (including non-steroidal anti-inflammatory drugs, sulphasalazine). Possible association with hepatitis C infection.

Prognosis
Unlike the cutaneous disease that resolves after 18–24 months, oral lichen planus is more persistent. Atrophic and erosive causes may progress to malignancy in about 2% of cases.

Management options
Withdrawal of precipitating drugs if this is the suspected cause.

Bullous Lesions

PEMPHIGUS VULGARIS
This is a rare disease that affects both sexes equally. Oral involvement occurs in 50% of patients. Fluid-filled bullae burst to leave painful shallow ulcers that resolve over weeks or months. The disease is relapsing and remitting. Antibodies to intraepithelial antigens can be detected. The key histological feature is acantholytic cells and the bullae form from suprabasal layers. Treatment: systemic steroids with or without azathioprine are required indefinitely.

PEMPHIGOID
Pemphigoid is another rare skin disorder producing bullous lesions in the mouth. It is more common in men and affects an older age group than pemphigus. Sub-epithelial bullae

Bullous Lesions

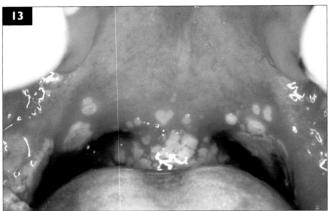

13 Candida infection – white plaques on the palate.

form as the epithelium detaches from the lamina propria; the bullae then rupture to leave ulcers. The condition may involve mouth, or other mucous membranes and the eye.

In treatment, in addition to steroids, dapsone may be helpful.

ERYTHEMA MULTIFORME

Occurs at all ages, and is more common in men. In its severest form it produces painful mucosal erosions and ulcers in the oral cavity. Oral involvement can occur in the absence of skin lesions, making the diagnosis difficult, and it must be differentiated from other bullous diseases. Management consists of withdrawing the precipitating drug if it can be identified.

Treatment: tetracycline mouthwashes and steroids.

HERPETIC GINGIVITIS

Herpetic gingivitis occurs in young children. There may be systemic illness with fever, sore throat and lymphadenopathy, followed by vesicle formation throughout the mouth. These vesicles ulcerate, coalesce and form large confluent areas of shallow ulceration.

Treatment is symptomatic: tetracycline mouthwashes to hinder secondary bacterial infection, and aciclovir for severe disease.

INFECTIVE GINGIVITIS (SYNONYM VINCENT'S INFECTION)

Bacterial infection of the gingival membrane can produce haemorrhagic gingival ulceration.

This may affect all ages, but is more common in smokers. Mixed organisms – largely mouth flora – are responsible, including Gram-negative anaerobes. Poor dental hygiene is important in the aetiopathogenesis. Severe disease occurs in immunocompromised patients. Patients complain of pain, bleeding gums, halitosis, regional lymphadenopathy and sometimes fever.

Prevention: involves careful oral toilet in debilitated and acutely ill patients at risk of infection. Treatment: antibiotics, dental cleaning and mouth washes are used to treat established infection.

CANDIDA (SYNONYM THRUSH)

A common oral commensal, but infection is unusual in the absence of predisposing factors such as antibiotics, systemic illness, immunocompromise and xerostomia (dry mouth, as in Sjögren's syndrome). White plaques are the most common manifestation (**13**), but painful glossitis (see **10**) and cheilitis (see **9**) are also seen. Palatal candida can present as a painful erythematous plaque in endentulous patients, sometimes in association with cheilitis.

A chronic hyperplastic form of candida with firm diffuse plaques of candida affects patients with AIDS as part of chronic mucocutaneous candidiasis.

Treatment: oral antifungals are sufficient for most patients, but systemic treatment is indicated for chronic mucocutaneous candidiasis.

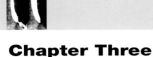
Oesophagus

Dysphagia is a potentially sinister symptom that requires investigation

Endoscopy is the most valuable form of investigation, but both barium radiology and motility studies may be helpful

Heartburn (pyrosis) due to reflux is common and may lead to oesophagitis. The relationship between hiatus hernia and reflux has been overemphasised in the past

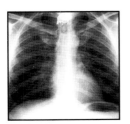
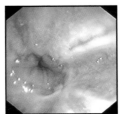
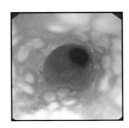
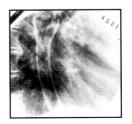

Anatomy/Histology

The oesophagus is a muscular tube which runs from the cricopharyngeal to the oesophagogastric junction. Anatomically, in the normal adult the oesophagogastric junction is approximately 38 cm from the incisor teeth.

Histologically, the mucosal lining comprises squamous epithelium, with surrounding layers of circular and longitudinal muscle. There are normal regenerative 'pegs' in the epithelium.

Investigating the Oesophagus

Endoscopy and barium radiology represent the primary means by which structural diseases of the oesophagus may be investigated.

RADIOLOGY

The classical radiological investigation of the oesophagus has been the barium swallow (**14**). Structural lesions such as ulcers and strictures are readily identified (**15**), and the technique is more sensitive than endoscopy in detecting extrinsic compression of the oesophagus. It is also better than endoscopy for the examination of oesophageal pouches, webs and rings and, since it is performed without sedation or instrumentation, it is safer than endoscopy.

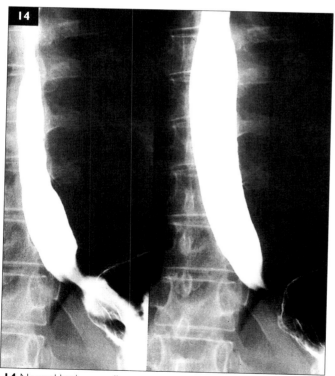

14 Normal barium swallow appearances.

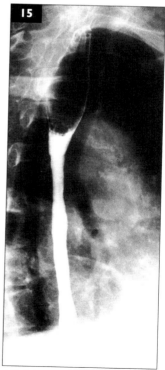

15 A long stricture in the oesophagus due to ingestion of caustic soda.

Investigating the Oesophagus

A plain chest X-ray may occasionally be helpful, revealing either the position of swallowed foreign bodies (16), or demonstrating gross dilatation of the oesophagus as in achalasia.

Mucosal disease

Barium radiology is less sensitive than endoscopy for small mucosal lesions and cannot reliably differentiate benign from malignant strictures. These should be assessed by endoscopic biopsy. Barium swallow should precede endoscopy in the investigation of dysphagia. The endoscopist is forewarned and this prevents the rare but potentially dangerous situation of intubating a pharyngeal pouch (potentially leading to perforation). It also indicates the level and likely nature of an obstructing lesion.

Reflux

Reflux of barium from stomach into the oesophagus can be demonstrated using barium, but since this can be provoked in many normal subjects it is not a reliable discriminator.

Motility

Swallowing disorders can be investigated using videofluoroscopy. Gross motility disorders affecting the body of the oesophagus, such as advanced achalasia or diffuse oesophageal spasm, can also be detected, but manometry is more sensitive.

ENDOSCOPY

Upper gastrointestinal endoscopy has revolutionised the practice of gastroenterology and has become routine (17). The small risk of complications is primarily related to the sedation that most patients are given, and to perforation and haemorrhage following instrumentation. The immediate advantage of endoscopy over barium radiology is the ability to take samples for histological and cytological assessment. This is mandatory in the assessment of oesophageal ulcers and strictures.

Reflux

Mucosal changes (ranging from subtle reddening to mucosal ulceration) can be detected in patients with gastro-oesophageal reflux disease, but in 30% of cases the endoscopic and histological appearances remain normal.

Motility

Although endoscopy is of no value in the diagnosis of motility disorders *per se*, patients with

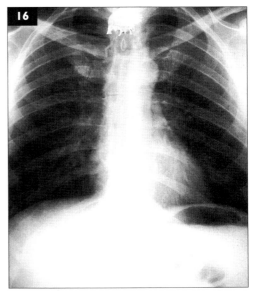

16 A foreign body (dental plate) lodged in the oesophagus.

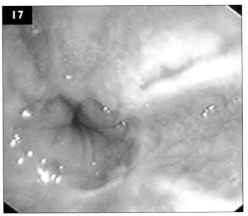

17 The oesophagogastric junction at endoscopy, with a streaky area of linear oesophagitis above it.

achalasia require endoscopy to exclude malignancy at the lower oesophagus or gastric cardia. Conversely, oesophageal motility disorders may be secondary to oesophagitis.

Investigating the Oesophagus

ENDOSCOPIC ULTRASOUND

High-resolution images of the oesophageal wall can be obtained using endoscopic ultrasound because the probe can be applied close to the lesion. Interfaces between layers in the gut wall are displayed as concentric rings. The technique has proved valuable in assessing local spread of oesophageal tumours.

OESOPHAGEAL PH STUDIES

Oesophageal pH monitoring detects reflux of acid into the oesophagus by use of a pH meter probe on a fine tube. The technique is unnecessary in most patients with gastro-oesophageal reflux disease and is reserved for patients with an atypical history, and those presenting with obscure chest pain. The frequency and duration of episodes of oesophageal reflux can be investigated by placing a pH electrode 5 cm above the lower oesophageal sphincter. The 'gold standard' is the percentage of time the intraoesophageal pH is <4 during a 24-hour period. This varies with age, but a value of >7% is abnormal in young people.

The sensitivity of the distal oesophagus to acid can be assessed by the Bernstein acid perfusion test. Saline or dilute acid is instilled into the mid-oesophagus via a fine-bore nasogastric tube, in order to determine whether acid perfusion reproduces symptoms, the subject being unaware of which is being perfused. This procedure may elucidate the cause of chest pain of obscure origin.

MANOMETRY

Cine or videofluoroscopy are used to assess oropharyngeal disorders where a food bolus cannot transit to the oesophagus, but motility disorders of the body of the oesophagus are best investigated by manometry (**18**). An oesophageal catheter records pressure at multiple levels in the oesophagus. The pressure records of spontaneous and swallowing-induced motor activity are recorded and analysed. Indications for oesophageal manometry include unexplained dysphagia, chest pain, and the pre-surgical evaluation of patients with oesophagitis.

OESOPHAGEAL SCINTIGRAPHY

Oesophageal function can also be investigated using oesophageal scintigraphy. Patients swallow a standard meal or drink containing a non-absorbable radiolabelled tracer which is detected by a gamma-camera. Motility disorders are detected by measuring the scintigraphic oesophageal transit, and scintigraphic tests of reflux generally correlate with oesophageal pH tests. This is quick, non-invasive and repeatable, and as the radiation dose is less than conventional radiology the technique is useful in longitudinal studies and paediatric patients.

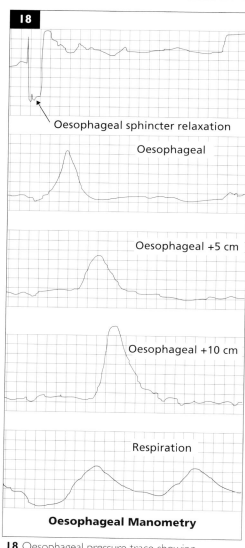

18

Oesophageal sphincter relaxation

Oesophageal

Oesophageal +5 cm

Oesophageal +10 cm

Respiration

Oesophageal Manometry

18 Oesophageal pressure trace showing progression of peristalsis.

Carcinoma of the Oesophagus

Definition
Primary cancer of the oesophagus.

Epidemiology and aetiology
Carcinoma of the oesophagus affects those aged over 65 primarily, and is more common in men than women. There are interesting geographic variations in the disease incidence, suggesting that environmental factors are important in its aetiology. Iran, China and parts of southern Africa have the highest rates. Alcohol and tobacco are independent aetiological factors that also act synergistically. Dietary factors include deficiency of trace elements and vitamins, intake of nitrites and nitrosamines and, in China, fungal contamination of foods. Other predisposing factors include Barrett's oesophagus, chronic oesophagitis, achalasia, peptic oesophageal ulceration and leucoplakia.

Pathophysiology
The macroscopic appearances range from ulcer to exophytic lesions and strictures. Squamous cell carcinoma is most common in the upper third of the oesophagus. Such carcinoma are generally radiosensitive and have a better prognosis than the adenocarcinomas, which are more frequent in the distal oesophagus. Adenocarcinomas arise in the columnar-lined mucosa of Barrett's oesophagus. The disease spreads locally, circumferentially in submucosal tissue, and into the adjacent mediastinal structures including trachea, pericardium and aorta. Lymphatic spread is common.

Clinical history
Dysphagia is the dominant symptom. Usually, this is relentlessly progressive, but in some patients the first manifestation of disease is complete dysphagia from an obstructing bolus of food. Regurgitation eventually occurs. Other symptoms may include pain on swallowing and cough. Cough may represent aspiration, or the development of an oesophagotracheal fistula. Recurrent laryngeal nerve palsy due to mediastinal spread causes hoarseness.

Physical examination
Examination is abnormal only in advanced disease. Secondary deposits may be palpable in supraclavicular lymph nodes. Mediastinal spread may lead to superior vena cava obstruction.

Laboratory and special investigations
Barium swallow is usually the first investigation of dysphagia (**19**). (This prevents unwittingly entering an undiagnosed pharyngeal pouch at endoscopy as the crico-oesophageal junction cannot always be visualised during intubation.)

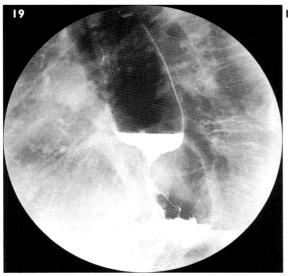

19 Barium swallow showing obstruction due to carcinoma of the oesophagus.

Carcinoma of the Oesophagus

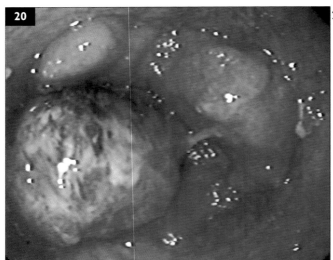

20 An oesophageal carcinoma in Barrett's oesophagus, almost obliterating the lumen.

Endoscopic biopsy and brushing of any suspicious lesions is mandatory (**20**).

Local spread can be assessed by endoscopic ultrasound if available. Thoracic computed tomography and cardiorespiratory assessment are indicated in those being considered for surgery.

Differential diagnosis
Gastric carcinoma spreading to the lower oesophagus may mimic oesophageal carcinoma. Lesions at the cardia may be misdiagnosed as achalasia when there is associated oesophageal dilatation. Peptic strictures may be indistinguishable from malignant strictures. Apparently benign 'peptic' strictures recurring soon after dilatation should be regarded with suspicion. A long history of reflux before the onset of dysphagia suggests benign peptic stricture, but biopsy remains mandatory.

Special forms
Patterson–Kelly syndrome (Plummer–Vinson syndrome).

In some women with long standing iron-deficiency anaemia, chronic inflammatory changes associated with hyperkeratinization occur in the hypopharynx. Cricopharyngeal spasm causes dysphagia. This syndrome is generally benign, but may be complicated by carcinoma.

Prognosis
The prognosis of oesophageal cancer is appalling, and most patients are dead within a year of diagnosis. The 5-year survival rate with surgery (in selected patients) is 5%.

Management
Surgery offers virtually the only prospect of cure. The best results are obtained in those patients with favourable tumours in the middle or lower thirds of the oesophagus treated by partial oesophagectomy or oesophagogastrectomy, respectively. This is a disease of the elderly and has high operative mortality rates. Surgery is only appropriate in adequately nourished patients with sufficient cardiorespiratory reserve. Lesions in the hypopharynx and upper third of the oesophagus are usually squamous and are managed by radiotherapy.

Dysphagia is a distressing symptom for patients and their relatives, so if surgery is impossible the principal aim is palliation of dysphagia. It can be relieved endoscopically or under radiological control by dilation (**21**), and oesophageal patency maintained by a stent (**22**). The potential complications include stent migration, blockage, and oesophageal perforation. Obstruction can be temporarily relieved by laser ablation if the facility is available. A cheaper alternative is endoscopic alcohol injection. Radiotherapy and stenting together may be appropriate for some squamous carcinomas.

Carcinoma of the Oesophagus

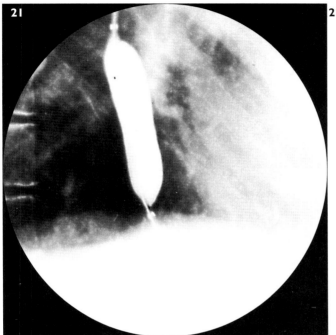

21 Dilatation of malignant stricture with a balloon under radiological control.

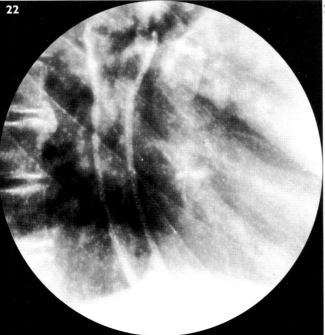

22 Passage of a rubber tube to maintain patency and allow swallowing.

Achalasia and other Primary Motility Disorders

Achalasia is defined as a condition of unknown aetiology associated with absent oesophageal peristalsis, and failure of relaxation of the lower oesophageal sphincter (LOS).

Epidemiology and aetiology
Achalasia is rare and affects both sexes equally. It occurs in adults of any age.

Pathophysiology
The key feature is ganglion loss from the myenteric neural plexus, which can be demonstrated histologically and is supported by pharmacological evidence of denervation. Progressive oesophageal dilatation arises from a combination of lack of peristalsis and failure of relaxation of the lower oesophageal sphincter. Diffuse thickening of the wall occurs from secondary changes in mucosal and smooth muscle layers.

Clinical history
Dysphagia This is progressive and – in contrast to most causes – characteristically presents with dysphagia for both liquids and solids from the outset.

Regurgitation Postprandial regurgitation may be described as vomiting by the patient, but it is generally effortless, without retching. Regurgitation on recumbency can lead to aspiration and repeated chest infections. Younger patients may complain of retrosternal chest pain.

Physical examination
There may be no physical signs.

Laboratory and special examinations
Barium studies in achalasia are variable. The oesophagus may be dilated and tortuous with a fluid level (sometimes visible on routine chest radiograph) (**23**), and 'bird's beak' tapering at the lower oesophageal sphincter. No peristalsis is seen on screening, and in advanced cases the gastric air bubble is absent. In manometric studies, resting lower oesophageal sphincter pressures may be elevated and relaxation is absent. Simultaneous pressure peaks (i.e. no propulsive contractions) are seen in the oesophageal body on swallowing.

Special forms
Mega-oesophagus associated with absent peristalsis occurs in amyloid. Paraneoplastic manifestations of

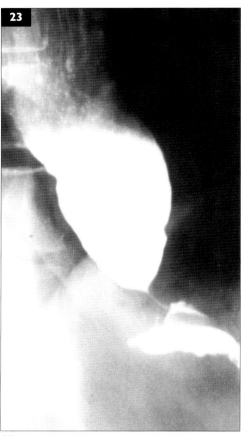

23 Achalasia of the oesophagus. Note the characteristic dilated oesophagus with fluid level, with a 'bird beak' tapering at the oesophagogastric junction.

carcinoma of the pancreas, stomach, and bronchus may mimic achalasia, but these patients have a shorter history of dysphagia (<1 year), and disproportionate weight loss. Secondary forms are seen in diabetic or alcoholic neuropathy, pseudo-obstruction and Chagas' disease (parasitic infection due to *Trypanosoma cruzi*).

Differential diagnosis
Carcinoma of the gastric cardia may both mimic and complicate achalasia. Endoscopy and biopsy

Achalasia and other Primary Motility Disorders

are therefore mandatory. Endoscopy is a frequent investigation in patients with dysphagia; although achalasia cannot be diagnosed this way it may be suspected when undigested food debris are seen in the oesophagus.

Prognosis
Squamous carcinoma may arise in the dilated segment. Respiratory complications may arise from aspiration.

Management
Medical therapy is unsatisfactory, but the lower oesophageal sphincter pressure may be reduced with isosorbide dinitrate or calcium antagonists. Better symptom control is achieved by disrupting the circular muscle fibres – either pneumatic dilation or surgical myotomy using a modified Heller's procedure (longitudinal slit through oesophageal muscle or cardia).

Abnormal peristalsis in the absence of mucosal lesion is seen in other conditions as well as achalasia.

DIFFUSE OESOPHAGEAL SPASM
Epidemiology and aetiology
This is rare, but it occurs in patients aged over 50 years, and in both sexes.

Pathophysiology
Not known.

Clinical history
Patients complain principally of retrosternal chest pain, with the character and distribution of angina. In 50% of patients, episodes are precipitated by eating but may also occur nocturnally. Symptoms may deteriorate under emotional stress. Some patients also have dysphagia.

Physical examination
Normal.

Laboratory and special examinations
Manometric abnormalities are similar to achalasia, but are less marked. Simultaneous, high-amplitude 'tertiary' contractions seen in the middle third of oesophagus, with impaired lower oesophageal sphincter relaxation and high resting pressures. A variety of segmental non-peristaltic contractions are seen on barium examination. Oesophageal dilation and retained food debris are unusual.

Other forms
'Hypertensive lower oesophageal sphincter' syndrome This appears as elevated resting lower oesophageal sphincter tone, occurring alone or in association with 'nut-cracker' oesophagus (24) which describes abnormally high distal oesophageal contractions, presenting with angina-like chest pain.

'Irritable oesophagus' These patients have symptoms of non-cardiac chest pain that are caused at different times by either acid reflux or dysmotility. They can be identified by 24-hour intraoesophageal pH and pressure measurements.

Differential diagnosis
Angina presents with a similar pain. In patients with achalasia, dysphagia is the predominant symptom.

Prognosis and treatment
Sublingual glyceryl trinitrate will relieve the pain of oesophageal spasm. Myotomy or dilatation are rarely indicated. Management of 'irritable oesophagus' is generally unsatisfactory and treatment must be directed towards either the dysmotility or reflux as appropriate.

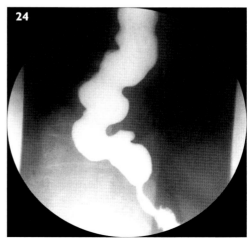

24 A nut-cracker oesophagus. Note the irregular, non-propulsive incoordinate contraction of the oesophagus.

Columnar-Lined Oesophagus (Barrett's Syndrome)

Definition
The presence of columnar epithelium extending as a cylinder or tongues more than 3 cm up the oesophagus above the gastric cardia. The epithelium is similar to gastric lining epithelium and replaces the normal stratified squamous epithelium.

Epidemiology and aetiology
The average age at presentation is 55 years and it is more common in men. Columnar lined oesophagus is found in up to 4% patients at endoscopy and in 20% of patients with oesophagitis.

Pathophysiology
The prevailing theory is that columnar lined oesophagus is due to gastro-oesophageal reflux. Chronic oesophageal mucosal inflammation and desquamation of the squamous epithelium occurs in the distal oesophagus. This is replaced by columnar lining epithelium as an adaptive response and thus the squamocolumnar junction migrates up the oesophagus. Gastro-oesophageal reflux is common in Barrett's patients, which supports this view.

Clinical history
Symptoms are usually due to the associated gastro-oesophageal reflux and oesophagitis.

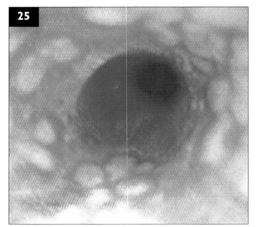

25 Barrett's oesophagus. The pink (columnar) epithelium extends way above the oesophagogastric junction, encircling islands of paler squamous (oesophageal) epithelium.

Physical examination
There are no physical signs.

Laboratory and special examinations
The diagnosis is suspected at endoscopy. Normally, the demarcation between pink–grey squamous epithelium and salmon-red columnar epithelium forms an irregular ring at the cardia called the ora serrata or 'Z' line. In the columnar-lined oesophagus, this migrates proximally as a cylinder, with islands of pink squamous mucosa or long irregular tongues of columnar mucosa rising into the oesophagus from the cardia (**25**). Endoscopic mucosal biopsies must be taken at multiple sites. This is to confirm the gastric columnar epithelium and detect dysplasia. *Helicobacter pylori* infection of the gastric metaplasia may also be found.

Special forms
Dysplasia and adenocarcinoma arise in the specialised metaplastic mucosa that occurs just above the squamocolumnar junction.

Differential diagnosis
Columnar-lined oesophagus lacks the rugae of stomach mucosa, which distinguishes it from sliding hiatus herniae. In practice, a more common error is to overlook the diagnosis of Barrett's syndrome, since the colour change from the pink squamous mucosa to the salmon-coloured columnar epithelium can be subtle.

Prognosis
There is an increased risk of developing adenocarcinoma. Estimates for the increased risk range between 30–100 times that in age-matched controls. Some authorities believe that 'short-segment' Barrett's is the principal origin of adenocarcinoma of the lower oesophagus.

Management
Gastro-oesophageal reflux and oesophagitis are treated conventionally. As yet, there is no firm evidence that proton pump inhibitors or surgery induce regression of the lesion, or reduce the risk of progression to adenocarcinoma.

Follow-up endoscopic screening is only worthwhile if the patient is prepared to accept oesophageal resection if high-grade dysplasia is detected. The economic benefit of surveillance is unclear.

Oesophageal Infections

CANDIDA

Candidal oesophagitis can be asymptomatic or cause oesophageal pain that is either persistent or occurs when swallowing (odynophagia). Like candidal infection elsewhere, it is more common in patients with diabetes, in patients receiving broad-spectrum antibiotic therapy, or corticosteroid treatment. It also occurs in the debilitated (including alcoholism) and immunosuppressed (including AIDS when pharyngeal plaques are sometimes seen).

Examinations/investigations

Nodular plaques of candida can be seen on barium swallow or generalised ulceration may be visualised (26). At endoscopy, white plaques of candida are seen on hyperaemic mucosa.

Diagnosis

This can be confirmed from biopsies or brushings.

Management

Treatment is by antifungals, e.g. nystatin or amphotericin, given orally.

HERPETIC OESOPHAGITIS

Herpetic oesophagitis is most common in the immunocompromised but has been reported in healthy people. It causes small vesicles and confluent superficial ulceration. Characteristic eosinophilic inclusions are seen on biopsy.

CYTOMEGALOVIRUS OESOPHAGITIS

Cytomegalovirus (CMV) is another cause of ulceration in the oesophagus and upper gastrointestinal tract in the immunocompromised. An 'owl's eye' nuclear inclusion is diagnostic on histopathological examination.

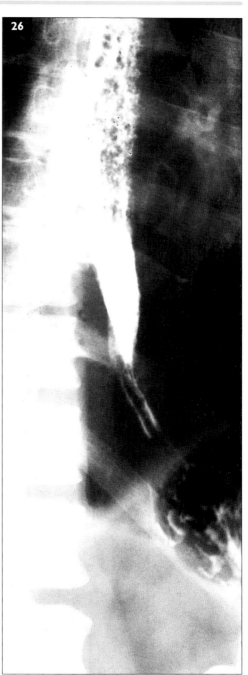

26 Oesophageal candidiasis – irregular filling defects due to plaques of candida.

Oesophageal Varices

Definition
Oesophageal varices are defined as dilated intramural oesophageal veins. They are portosystemic venous communications and the direct result of portal hypertension (**27, 28**). Oesophageal varices can bleed and this makes them the most important manifestation of portal hypertension in clinical practice.

Pathophysiology
Normally, all the blood delivered to the liver by the portal venous system returns through the liver to the systemic circulation via the hepatic veins. With cirrhosis, and when the portal venous system is obstructed, this does not occur. Portal venous pressure rises and portovenous shunts open to enable venous blood to return to the systemic circulation via alternative routes (**29**).

Clinical history
The patient may have a prior history of bleeding oesophageal varices and of the underlying liver disease.

Physical examination
Physical signs of portal hypertension include splenomegaly, dilated abdominal veins (flow is away from the umbilicus), and rectal varices. Since the principal cause of portal hypertension is liver cirrhosis, evidence of this is generally present.

Laboratory and special investigations
Oesophageal varices can be diagnosed by barium swallow and can be accentuated by a reverse Valsalva manoeuvre. Endoscopy is preferable as the size of the varices, and the presence of red signs (suggesting imminent risk of bleeding) can then be assessed.

Other features of portal hypertension may be seen, e.g. gastric fundal varices or portal hypertensive gastropathy. This is another manifestation of portal hypertension, with a range of endoscopic appearances from a mosaic 'snakeskin' pattern through to 'watermelon' stomach. Bleeding is usually chronic and self-limiting, but patients can become anaemic.

The investigation of portal hypertension includes assessment of portal vein patency by Doppler ultrasound or angiography, and appropriate investigation of the liver. Portal pressures can be assessed indirectly by the difference between the wedged and free hepatic venous pressures, but this approach is not routine and is usually only carried out in specialised centres.

Special forms
Portal hypertension can occur in the absence of liver disease, for instance, portal vein thrombosis due to neonatal umbilical sepsis or instrumentation. Splenic vein thrombosis also causes portal hypertension, especially gastric fundal varices and is a complication of pancreatitis and blunt abdominal trauma (e.g. steering wheel injury in a road traffic accident). Other causes of non-cirrhotic portal hypertension include congenital hepatic fibrosis and hepatic schistosomiasis. The importance of these uncommon conditions is that liver function is preserved, and the prognosis after variceal haemorrhage is much better.

Differential diagnosis
Gastrointestinal bleeding in patients who have oesophageal varices is not always variceal. Peptic ulcers are more common in the cirrhotic population and these are said to be more difficult to heal with H_2 receptor antagonists. The gastric mucosa is also more sensitive to injury than normal.

Prognosis
Although only 30% of patients bleed from their oesophageal varices, the overall mortality rate for first bleed is around 50%. There are no reliable means of predicting which patients will bleed, but endoscopic signs are of some value. Larger varices (higher wall tension), varices with 'red signs' and patients with more severe underlying liver disease are at greatest risk.

Management
Prophylactic treatment In alcoholic cirrhosis, abstinence will reduce the size of varices. Portal pressure can be reduced pharmacologically by propranolol and to a lesser extent by oral nitrates. In order to reduce the risk of bleeding the pressure gradient must be <12 mmHg. There is no place for prophylactic sclerotherapy.

Bleeding The management of bleeding oesophageal varices (discussed in Chapter 10) involves prompt resuscitation and haemodynamic monitoring.

Oesophageal Varices

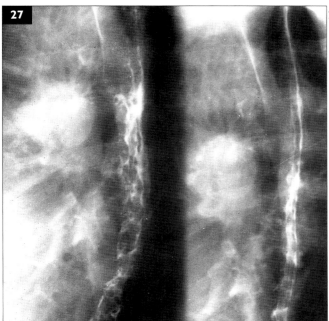

27 Oesophageal varices – these show as worm-like filling defects in the oesophagus on barium meal.

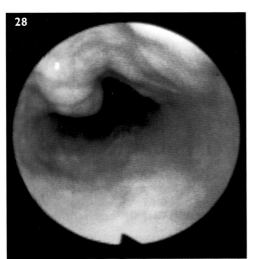

28 Oesophageal varices seen as varicose veins at endoscopy.

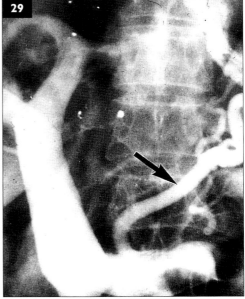

29 This angiogram shows the vascular anatomy of portal hypertension with (arrowed) a varix leaving the portal vein.

Oesophageal Varices

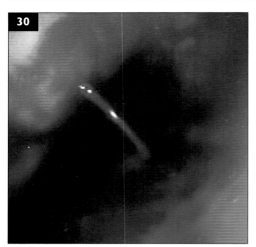

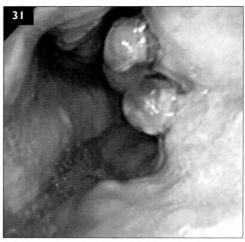

30 An oesophageal varix, bleeding.

31 Oesophageal varices which have just been treated by 'banding'; that is, placing a rubber band about them.

Variceal haemorrhage must be staunched by balloon tamponade, endoscopic sclerotherapy (**30**) or ligation (**31**) or pharmacological means. This includes drugs to cause acute reduction of portal pressure and blood flow using drugs such as somatostatin, vasopressin and their analogues.

The interventional radiological technique, transvenous intrahepatic portal-systemic shunting (TIPSS), directly lowers portal pressure by creating a direct shunt from portal to hepatic vein. Direct surgical procedures of oversewing or ligating varices, or (less common nowadays) creation of a surgical shunt between portal and systemic vessels, can also be used in emergencies.

Oesophageal Webs and Rings

Definition
Mucosal abnormalities are common in the oesophagus. Webs are folds of squamous mucosa that protrude into the lumen and may be found at all levels of the oesophagus (**32, 33**). Rings are circumferential, their upper surface is covered by stratified squamous epithelium and columnar epithelium occurs on the lower surface.

'Schatzki's ring' (**34, 35**) is the most commonly encountered, as a thin submucosal scar at the squamocolumnar junction.

Aetiology and pathophysiology
It is proposed that Schatzki's rings arise in response to chronic injury by gastro-oesophageal reflux.

Clinical history
Some patients have no symptoms and the diagnosis is made incidentally. Dysphagia is unusual if the lumen is more than 20 mm. However, sudden complete dysphagia can occur due to obstruction of a bolus of food – the so-called 'steak-house syndrome'.

Management
Symptomatic rings or webs can be dilated and anti-reflux measures instituted.

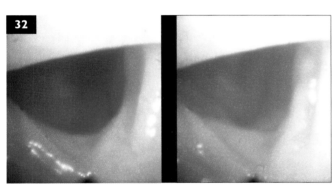

32 Web seen in the cricopharyngeal area.

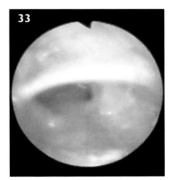

33 An oesophageal web at endoscopy.

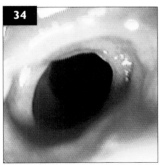

34 Oesophageal (Schatzki's) ring.

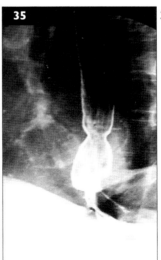

35 Schatzki's ring visualised by barium swallow.

Diverticula and Pouches

Definition
Oesophageal diverticula are outpouchings of one or more layers of the oesophageal wall. They occur at three levels in the oesophagus – pharyngeal (immediately above the cricopharyngeus muscle), mid-oesophageal and epiphrenic (just above the diaphragm).

Pharyngeal pouches Also known as Zenker's diverticulum, these are the most important type as they cause dysphagia and aspiration (**36, 37**).

Mid-oesophageal diverticula These are rarely symptomatic and arise either because of oesophageal dysmotility (pulsion) or because of mediastinal traction from tuberculosis (**38**).

Epiphrenic diverticula These occur in association with other diseases affecting oesophageal motility.

Aetiology, epidemiology and pathophysiology
Pharyngeal pouches are uncommon and affect the elderly. The diverticula arise in the midline posteriorly between the inferior constrictor and the cricopharyngeus muscles. It enlarges as a thin-walled sac, typically deviating to the left side of the neck. The aetiology may be failure of relaxation during swallowing due to primary cricopharyngeal dysfunction, sometimes referred to as 'cricopharyngeal achalasia'. There is an association with hiatus herniae.

Clinical history
Patients present with dysphagia, regurgitation and weight loss. There is a risk of aspiration.

Physical examination
Large pouches can sometimes be palpated in the neck after food has been eaten.

Laboratory and special examinations
Barium swallow is the most appropriate initial investigation (see **37**). The pouch appears as a 'teapot spout'. Cine-radiology is helpful in early cases. Endoscopy should be performed cautiously as the cricopharyngeal area is often a 'blind' region during intubation and this can be dangerous.

Prognosis
Complicating squamous carcinoma have been reported rarely.

Management
Surgical options include cricopharyngeal myotomy, with or without excision of the pouch.

Diverticula and Pouches

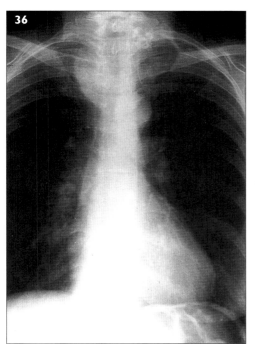

36 Chest X-ray showing outline of pharyngeal pouch in right upper mediastinum.

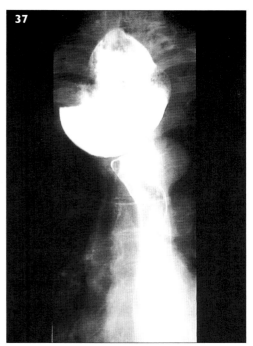

37 Barium swallow showing pharyngeal pouch.

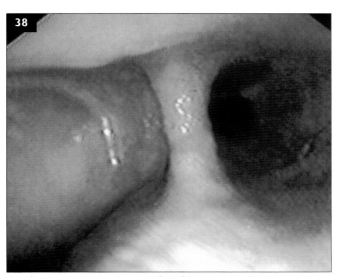

38 Oesophageal diverticulum (fluid-filled on the left).

Hiatus Hernia

Definition
A hiatus hernia occurs when part of the stomach leaves its normal anatomical position in the abdomen and enters the thorax. There are two forms: axial (sliding) and paraoesophageal (rolling).

Epidemiology
Axial hiatus hernias are common and are usually present in up to 50% of 50-year-olds. Paraoesophageal hernias are less common and present at a later age.

Pathophysiology
Axial (sliding) hiatus hernia
The normal relationship between oesophagus and stomach is maintained, but the cardia is displaced into the thorax (39, 40). Lower oesophageal sphincter function is compromised by herniation and gastro-oesophageal reflux occurs. Transient physiological herniation when the oesophagus shortens is normal, occurring during vomiting. It has been suggested that contraction of longitudinal oesophageal smooth muscle underlies the pathogenesis of axial hiatus hernia. As stimulation of intra-abdominal structures initiates oesophageal smooth muscle contraction, this may explain the clinical associations between gallstone disease and hiatus hernia.

Paraoesophageal hiatus hernia   In paraoesophageal hiatus hernia the gastric fundus herniates lateral to the cardia through a diaphragmatic weakness due to failed closure of the lateral pleuroperitoneal canal.

Clinical history
Most patients with axial hiatus hernias are asymptomatic. Classical symptoms are heartburn (pyrosis), acid regurgitation and water-brash. Dysphagia indicates oesophagitis or the development of stricture. Severe reflux can lead to pulmonary aspiration.

   The classical symptom of paraoesophageal hernias is dysphagia that changes with posture. Heartburn is not a feature. Most patients present with vague upper gastrointestinal symptoms or the hernia is noted as an incidental finding on chest radiograph. Anaemia from intractable ulceration at the neck of the hernia is common ('riding-ulcer'). There is a serious risk of strangulation, obstruction of the herniated stomach, and gastric volvulus.

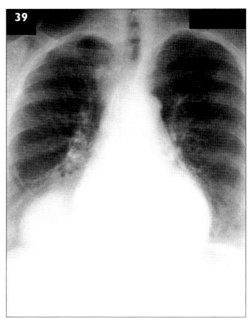

39 Plain X-ray showing hiatus hernia adjacent to right heart border.

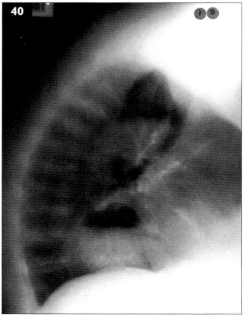

40 Lateral X-ray of hiatus hernia showing fluid level in stomach within chest.

Hiatus Hernia

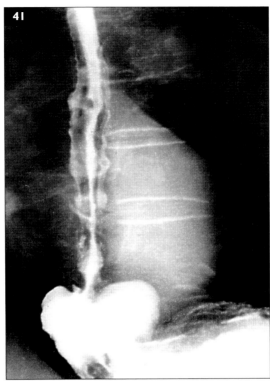

41 Hiatus hernia, showing protrusion of upper portion of stomach through the diaphragm.

Physical examination
This is usually normal.

Laboratory and special examinations
Mild reflux symptoms need not be investigated. Barium radiology will demonstrate both paraoesophageal and axial hiatus hernia (**41**). Axial hiatus hernia can usually be seen at endoscopy, but small hernia will be reduced by intubating the stomach and so escape notice. Negotiating a large axial hiatus hernia can be difficult at endoscopy.

Management
Asymptomatic axial hiatus hernias require no treatment.

If treatment is required, the general management approach is that for reflux. Those with mild reflux symptoms are advised to avoid stooping, to avoid tight-fitting garments, and to sleep with head of the bed elevated. Frequent light meals are better tolerated than large meals and in some patients specific foods induce symptoms – these should be avoided. The value of these measures is questionable and largely untested. Patients should be advised that smoking reduces the lower oesophageal tone and is a mucosal irritant and liable to worsen symptoms. Increasingly, severe symptoms should be managed with alginates and antacids, acid suppression with H_2 receptor antagonist or proton pump inhibitors as a stepped approach as for gastro-oesophageal reflux disease (GORD).

The incidence and severity of complications in paraoesophageal hiatus hernia means that all patients should be considered for surgical repair. However, because of the greater age and frailty of these patients this is often impractical.

Gastro-Oesophageal Reflux Disease and Oesophagitis

Definition
The terminology is confused. Reflux of gastric contents is a normal occurrence postprandially and is only considered abnormal if it gives rise to symptoms – referred to as gastro-oesophageal reflux disease (GERD in the USA, GORD in the UK).

Oesophagitis refers to the subsequent oesophageal mucosal injury that occurs in a minority of patients (**42**).

Epidemiology and aetiology
Up to one-third of the population have symptoms of reflux, but only a minority have oesophagitis. Apart from during pregnancy when it is a common complaint, symptoms are more severe in those aged over 50 – possibly reflecting an age-related decline in oesophageal motor function. Smoking and obesity are aggravating factors and non-steroidal anti-inflammatory drugs (NSAIDs) (including aspirin) are definite aetiological factors; they may act by reducing mucosal defence against injury.

Helicobacter pylori infection does not seem to play a significant role.

Pathophysiology
Intraoesophageal pH is <4 for a greater percentage of the time in patients compared with controls and this is correlated with the degree of mucosal injury. Two abnormalities are commonly detected in patients:
- Gastric juice refluxes into the oesophagus during episodes when lower oesophageal sphincter tone is transiently reduced.
- Oesophageal clearance of the refluxate is impaired.

There is controversy as to the importance of sliding hiatus hernia to the pathogenesis of GORD. Movement of the lower oesophageal sphincter to the thorax from the abdomen means it is subject to negative intrathoracic pressures and the protective effect of coordinated contractions of the diaphragmatic crurae are lost. These abnormalities increase the likelihood of reflux episodes on straining. The quality of the refluxate is rarely important unless the patient has Zollinger–Ellison syndrome (gross gastric hyperacidity stimulated by a neuroendocrine tumour releasing the hormone gastrin). Bile is very irritant and increases oesophageal injury but, except after gastric surgery, biliary reflux is uncommon

The histological changes in the mucosa range from mild inflammation to complete denuding of the squamous epithelium.

Clinical history
The most distinctive symptom is heartburn. Typically, it is experienced postprandially and is exacerbated by large, fatty meals. Some patients associate symptoms with particular foods. Bloating, nausea, anorexia, regurgitation and odynophagia also occur.

Dysphagia occurs either as a consequence of a secondary motility disorder or, less commonly, because of a peptic stricture (**43**). Respiratory symptoms arising from oesphagopharyngeal reflux are rare, but it may underlie some cases of asthma.

Physical examination
There are no physical signs.

Gastro-Oesophageal Reflux Disease and Oesophagitis

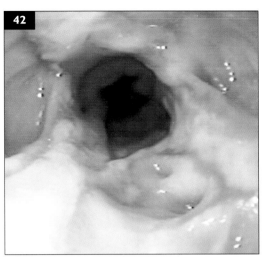

42 Reflux oesophagitis with ulceration and scarring.

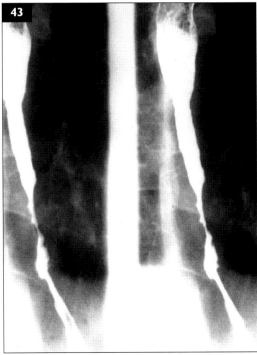

43 Extensive reflux oesophageal stricture seen on barium study.

Gastro-Oesophageal Reflux Disease and Oesophagitis

Laboratory and special investigations
In a young patient with typical symptoms investigation is unnecessary. The mucosal damage is usually confined to the distal 5 cm of the oesophagus, and is best assessed at endoscopy(**42**, **44–46**). Oesophagitis can be graded, lesions brushed and biopsied and the presence of Barrett's columnar-lined oesophagus determined.

Oesophageal pH monitoring (**47**) is reserved for the patient with atypical symptoms, obscure chest pains and in the investigation of reflux in relationship to respiratory symptoms.

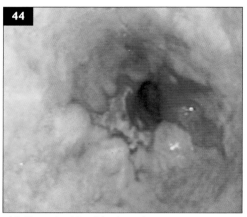

44 Oesophagitis with ulceration.

Differential diagnosis
The diagnosis is usually straightforward. Other causes of distal oesophageal ulceration include CMV, herpes and candida in the immunocompromised.

Strictures (**43**, **45**, **46**) associated with oesophagitis need to be differentiated from malignant strictures.

Prognosis
For most patients, GORD is a chronic condition with intermittent exacerbations of symptoms. Those patients with severe circumferential oesophagitis are at risk of peptic stricture and columnar-lined oesophagus.

Management
The aim of treatment is symptomatic relief and the prevention of complications. This requires a stepped approach. Patients with minimal symptoms and no mucosal damage should be treated conservatively by avoiding precipitating factors, and should lose weight. Preventing reflux at night by elevating the foot of the bed may help. Acid suppression with H_2 receptor antagonists and prokinetic agents such as cisapride will help some patients, progressing to proton pump inhibitor treatment for those with severe disease. Many patients will not achieve adequate symptom relief without proton pump inhibitors. Anti-reflux surgery is an option for patients with refractory symptoms, stricture, haemorrhage (rare) or respiratory complications.

Peptic strictures can be dilated either endoscopically or by using a balloon under radiographic control if symptomatic dysphagia occurs (**45**).

Gastro-Oesophageal Reflux Disease and Oesophagitis

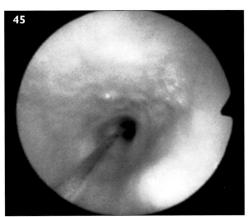

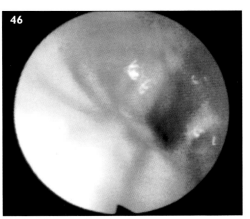

45 A peptic stricture caused by reflux into the oesophagus, with a guidewire passed through (before dilatation).

46 Peptic oesophageal stricture.

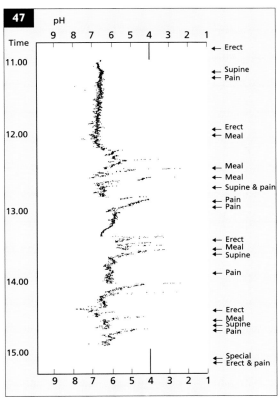

47 24-hour oesophageal pH monitoring, showing frequent episodes of reflux (low pH).

Stomach and Duodenum

Inflammatory diseases and neoplasia dominate gastric pathology. Neoplasia is very rare in the duodenum

Helicobacter pylori can cause acute and chronic gastritis, and predisposes to gastric and duodenal ulceration, gastric atrophy, and gastric cancer

Endoscopy is the predominant diagnostic modality

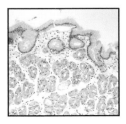
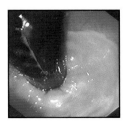
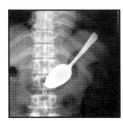
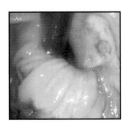

Stomach: Anatomy and Histology

The stomach extends from the oesophagogastric junction below the diaphragm to the pylorus (gastroduodenal junction), the latter being fixed to the peritoneum. The oesophagogastric junction may be mobile (hiatus hernia). The anatomical borders are the lesser and greater curves, but the body of the stomach is mobile and can be distorted. The stomach may be divided into the cardia, fundus, body and antrum (**48,49**). The acid-producing mucosa is located predominantly in the body.

Histology
As in all other parts of the intestine, layers of wall of gut consist of:
- Mucosa.
- Muscularis mucosa (thin layer of poorly organised muscle).
- Submucosa (connective tissue).
- Circular muscle fibres.
- Longitudinal muscle fibres.
- Outer serosal lining.

The gastric mucosa is specialised for acid production, which occurs in pit-like glands lined with acid-producing cells (parietal cells) (**50**). These cells contain the proton pump. A specialised area of the glands is responsible for regenerating cells, which migrate to reform surface epithelium. The luminal surface of the gastric mucosa is covered with a mucous layer, which traps a protective layer of bicarbonate to protect mucosal cells from acid.

Gastric antral histology is different in that there is no acid production. The antrum is responsible for the control of acid production, with a high concentration of gastrin-producing cells in the submucosa. Stimulation of gastrin following an increase in gastric pH (due to food ingestion) leads to acid release from parietal cells. When the stomach is empty and the pH falls, gastrin production is switched off. Circular and longitudinal smooth muscle activity is coordinated to allow peristaltic waves to pass the food through to the gastrointestinal tract.

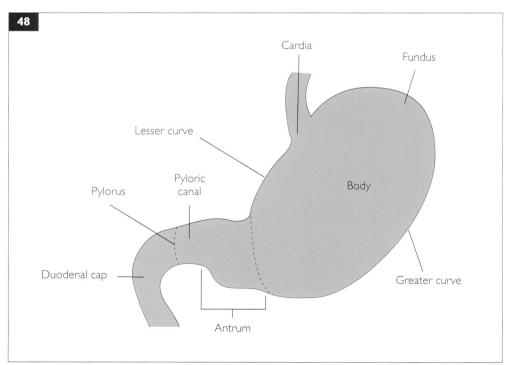

48   Anatomical areas of the stomach.

Stomach: Anatomy and Histology

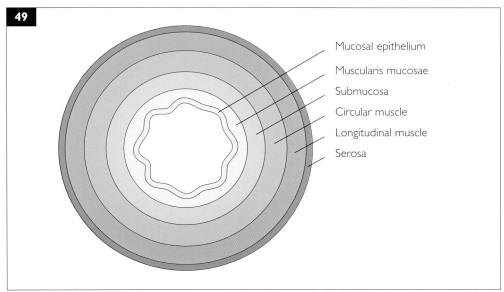

Mucosal epithelium

Muscularis mucosae

Submucosa

Circular muscle

Longitudinal muscle

Serosa

49 layers of the stomach (or intestinal) wall.

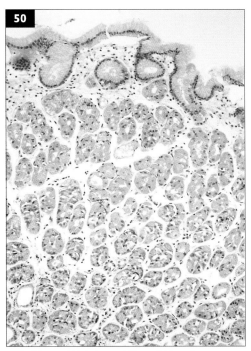

50 Normal histology of the acid-bearing area of stomach.

Investigation of the Stomach

Upper gastrointestinal symptoms are common in the general population, but they lack specificity and discriminate poorly between functional disease and organic pathology. Consequently, many patients are referred for upper gastrointestinal tract investigation.

ENDOSCOPY

This is the most common investigation (**51**). Endoscopy is more sensitive than radiology in detecting mucosal changes, but the chief advantage of endoscopy is that samples from any lesion can be sent for histological or cytological assessment and infection of the mucosa (by *H. pylori*) can be assessed. Also, the use of endoscopic ultrasound is increasing and has proved especially useful in the diagnosis of submucosal lesions, in differentiating these from extrinsic compression, and in assessing the local spread or recurrence of gastric tumours.

There are attendant risks from sedation (especially in patients with concurrent cardiorespiratory disease), and perforation or haemorrhage following instrumentation. Although the risk is small in diagnostic endoscopy (mortality of the order of 1:10 000), it is higher in therapeutic procedures.

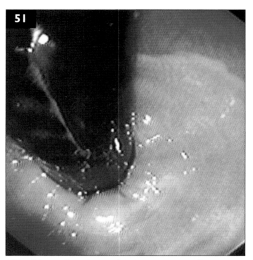

51 Normal endoscopic appearances of stomach.

Postoperative stomach

Except for the immediate postoperative phase, the complications of the post-surgical stomach such as stomal ulceration, gastritis, oesophagitis, bezoar formation and tumour recurrence are best assessed endoscopically.

Gastrointestinal bleeding

Emergency endoscopy in patients with upper gastrointestinal bleeding will identify the cause, and in cases of peptic ulcer bleeding, endoscopic criteria will assist in stratifying the risk of rebleeding. As well as accurate diagnosis, endoscopic treatment of the bleeding lesion is possible (for example by sclerotherapy, injection of alcohol, or heat or laser treatment).

RADIOLOGY

The barium meal examination is excellent for detecting anatomical variations such as large hiatus hernias or chronic gastric volvulus that can be bewildering to the endoscopist. Double-contrast studies are now routine and can delineate mucosal lesions such as polyps, erosions and ulcers. Although benign and malignant ulcers can be separated using radiological criteria, this is not sufficiently sensitive and all gastric ulcers must be assessed histologically by multiple repeated biopsies at endoscopy.

Postoperative stomach

Radiological assessment is useful to investigate the early complications in the postoperative stomach. Examples include anastomotic leakage or postoperative obstruction which are best investigated with water-soluble contrast radiology.

Gastrointestinal bleeding

The presence of lesions potentially causing upper gastrointestinal haemorrhage can be detected using contrast radiology, but whether or not they are the source of blood loss cannot be determined. Small erosions require sensitive double-contrast techniques.

Motility

Barium meal examination is better than endoscopy at detecting loss of antral peristalsis and antral narrowing. This occurs in diffuse infiltrative processes such as linitis plastica from gastric carcinoma or lymphoma, chronic granulomatous diseases (Crohn's, tuberculosis,

Investigation of the Stomach

sarcoidosis and syphilis) and amyloid. These can be missed at endoscopy unless a full-thickness or snare biopsy is taken.

Gastroparesis (loss of motility due to autonomic neuropathy in diabetics) and slow gastric emptying can be detected by barium meal, but are best quantitated by scintigraphy.

GASTRIC SCINTIGRAPHY
Some estimate of gastric emptying can be made by barium meal, and gastric stasis is suggested by the finding of food residue in a fasted stomach at endoscopy; however, this is best studied by gastric scintigraphy. Scintigraphic studies use a gamma-camera to follow the progress of a standard meal containing a non-absorbable tracer (52). After gastric surgery, very rapid gastric emptying can occur and in some cases food transits the stomach in 5 minutes. In most patients, symptoms improve during the first 18 months postoperatively and, by using this technique, clinical progress can be monitored.

GASTRIC ACID SECRETION
In the past, gastric acid secretion was frequently studied in the investigation of patients with pernicious anaemia (who have achlorhydria) and to assess acid secretion following vagotomy for peptic ulceration. Today, it is used in research and sometimes in the investigation of suspected Zollinger–Ellison syndrome.

Gastric contents are aspirated via a nasogastric tube in a fasted subject. Basal, unstimulated secretion is measured over 1 hour with four, 15-minute samples. Gastric acid secretion is then stimulated with intravenous pentagastrin and further samples collected. Stimulated secretion is expressed as either maximal acid output (the total 1-hour acid output after pentagastrin) or peak acid output (twice the sum of the two highest acid outputs over two consecutive 15-minute collections). The maximal and peak acid output are a measure of parietal cell mass, which is higher in men than women. It is increased in Zollinger–Ellison syndrome and is lower following antrectomy.

ZOLLINGER–ELLISON SYNDROME
This is a rare condition caused by a gastrin-secreting tumour (generally in the pancreas or duodenum, 53). It can be part of the multiple endocrine neoplasia (MEN) 1 syndrome, a genetic syndrome in which gastrin-secreting

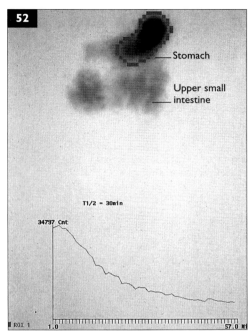

52 A technetium labelled meal, showing gradual emptying of the isotope from the stomach. The rate of loss can be quantified. In this example the t½ (time to half-emptying of the stomach) is 30 minutes.

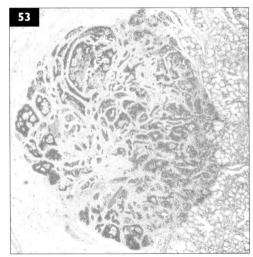

53 A gastrinoma in the wall of the duodenum, demonstrating how small they can be, but still responsible for devastating hyperacidity.

Investigation of the Stomach

tumours are associated with pituitary tumours (e.g. prolactinoma) and hyperparathyroidism. Patients present with multiple peptic ulcers extending into the distal duodenum and jejunum as a consequence of gastrin-driven acid secretion. Diarrhoea is reported in up to one-third of patients – probably reflecting pH-dependent inhibition of pancreatic lipases.

Pathology and pathophysiology
The tumours are often multiple, most often in the pancreas, and in two-thirds of patients the tumours are malignant. Basal acid and stimulated acid secretion is raised, but there is overlap into the reference range. Hyper-gastrinaemia is found and, unlike normal subjects, intravenous infusion of the hormone secretin augments serum gastrin levels.

Treatment
Acid hypersecretion is controlled medically by high-dose proton pump inhibitor treatment and, if possible, the primary tumour is excised surgically. Tumour localisation can be problematic and may require angiography and intraoperative ultrasound.

Gastritis

Gastritis is inflammation of the gastric mucosa. Until recently, classification has been contentious but an international working party has recently proposed a new scheme. The purpose was to incorporate endoscopic and biopsy findings and to recognise the bacterium *Helicobacter pylori* as the principal cause of chronic, non-immune gastritis. This so-called 'Sydney classification' makes a distinction between acute, chronic and special forms of gastritis and has a histological division and endoscopic division. The histological division covers inflammation (chronic inflammatory cells), activity (neutrophils), atrophy (diminution of gastric glands), intestinal metaplasia and the presence of *H. pylori*. The endoscopic division describes the endoscopic appearance of the mucosa.

ACUTE GASTRITIS
Definition
Gastric mucosal injury leading to an acute inflammation with or without ulceration.

Pathophysiology
There are several causes:
- Direct gastric mucosal injury can be caused by alcohol, corrosives, drugs and irradiation.
- Stress ulceration is associated with hypovolaemia, major trauma, sepsis, multi-organ failure, head injury (Cushing's ulcer) and burns (Curling's ulcer). Stress ulcers arise as a result of impaired gastric mucosal blood flow.

- Bacterial infection such as acute food poisoning (e.g. *Staphylococcus aureus* toxins).

Clinical history and examination
Patients complain of abdominal pain, anorexia, nausea, retching and haematemesis.

Laboratory and special examinations
The mucosa is erythematous and congested at endoscopy. Erosions (mucosal lesions without depth) (**54**), ulceration and haemorrhage (**55**) are also seen.

Special forms
Acute corrosive gastritis This is a serious condition following ingestion of acids, alkali or other necrotising agents. Patients can become shocked and gastric necrosis can ensue. Management is with nasogastric aspiration, acid suppression and surgery if necrosis develops.

Acute phlegmonous gastritis This is severe purulent bacterial infection of the full thickness of the gastric wall caused by Gram-positive cocci or coliforms. The condition is rare, usually affecting patients with pre-existing mucosal disease of the stomach. The patient is systemically ill with an acute abdomen, pyrexia, leucocytosis and purulent vomiting. Management is with anti-biotics, rehydration and surgery.

Differential diagnosis
Differentiation from other forms of gastric inflammation (e.g. chronic ulceration) and chronic gastritis is important.

Gastritis

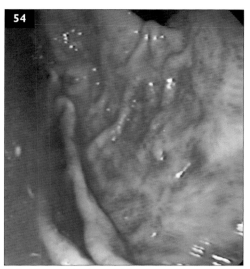

54 Haemorrhagic gastritis.

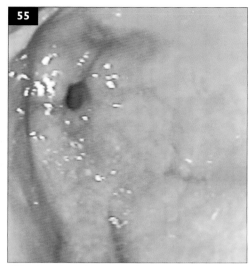

55 Antral erosions at endoscopy.

Prognosis
The prognosis depends on the cause.

Management
Prompt resuscitation, correction of organ failure and treatment of sepsis is essential. Prophylactic measures should be instituted in patients at risk of acute stress ulceration (e.g. patients in intensive care units). Various approaches have included acid suppression with H_2 receptor antagonists, antacids and sucralfate.

CHRONIC GASTRITIS
Definition
Chronic gastritis encompasses the various conditions associated with chronic inflammatory infiltrate in the gastric mucosa.

Epidemiology
Histological features of chronic gastritis are found in up to 50% of normal asymptomatic people.

Aetiology
The major cause of chronic gastritis is now recognised as *H. pylori* infection, which is responsible for around 80% of all cases. Idiopathic chronic gastritis accounts for 10–15% and autoimmune chronic gastritis about 5%. Specific, rarer, forms such as granulocytic (Crohn's, sarcoidosis, tuberculosis and syphylis)

eosinophilic and rugal hypertrophic gastritis account for the remainder.

Pathophysiology
H. pylori-associated chronic gastritis is discussed on pages 49–51.

In autoimmune chronic gastritis, parietal cell destruction is assumed to be a consequence of lymphocytic infiltration. Recently, the proton pump has been shown to be one of the antigens recognised by parietal cell autoantibodies. As the corpus mucosa becomes atrophic and thinned in advanced disease, gastric acidity falls. As a result, gastrin-producing neuroendocrine cells in the autoimmune (G-cells) respond by high levels of gastrin, leading to hypergastrinaemia.

Clinical history
The presence of gastritis is poorly correlated with symptomatic dyspepsia. Endoscopic duodenitis and active peptic ulcer disease are more closely linked.

Physical examination
There are usually no physical signs. Autoimmune chronic gastritis is often associated with other autoimmune diseases such as vitiligo, thyroid disorders, Addison's disease, type I diabetes mellitus, and signs of these may be evident.

Gastritis

Laboratory and special examinations

Endoscopy may show diffuse reddening or patchy abnormalities (**56**) but these findings are not specific. As the mucosa can be macroscopically normal in chronic gastritis, biopsy is essential for the diagnosis and to determine the cause. *H. pylori* is the most common cause of chronic gastritis and this should be sought by histology, culture or urease tests. Parietal cell autoantibodies are present in the serum in 90% of autoimmune chronic gastritis; intrinsic factor antibodies occur in the minority (<20%) who are likely to progress to pernicious anaemia. In established pernicious anaemia, serum vitamin B_{12} levels are low. Following ingestion of labelled vitamin B_{12}, <10% is excreted in the urine within 24 hours, but this is corrected when ingestion of B_{12} is repeated with intrinsic factor (Schilling test).

Special forms

Autoimmune chronic gastritis Autoimmune chronic gastritis causes an antral-sparing atrophic gastritis with hypergastrinaemia. Histologically, it is inactive (no polymorphonuclear leucocytes), unlike *H. pylori*-associated gastritis. There is an increased risk of epithelial dysplasia and gastric cancer (approximately three-fold). Hyperplastic and adenomatous gastric polyps are also more common. Rarely, multiple benign gastric carcinoid tumours may arise as a consequence of hypergastrinaemia, which stimulates proliferation of the enterochromaffin-like cells in the mucosa.

Differential diagnosis

Differentiate from acute gastritis and chronic ulceration.

Prognosis

The condition may predispose to gastric cancer, but is often asymptomatic and non-progressive.

Management

Treatment is symptomatic. Antacids, and acid suppression may help. *H. pylori* eradication is rarely symptomatically helpful (unless gastric or duodenal ulceration present). Whether *H. pylori* should be eradicated in an attempt to prevent subsequent development of gastric cancer is controversial. Pernicious anaemia is treated with injections of vitamin B_{12} (1000 µg every 2–3 months). Endoscopic surveillance for the early detection of gastric cancer in pernicious anaemia is controversial.

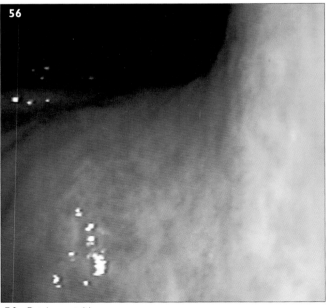

56 Patchy gastritis.

Helicobacter Pylori

Helicobacter pylori is now recognised as the major acquired factor in the aetiology of duodenal ulcer disease. This realisation has prompted a major reappraisal of the aetiology, pathophysiology, and management of peptic ulcer disease.

H. pylori is a curved or spiral flagellated, Gram-negative microaerophilic bacteria. Despite the original classification as *Campylobacter*-like, it has no relationship to these organisms and is not linked to *Campylobacter* infections elsewhere in the gastrointestinal tract. The specific features of *H. pylori* that allow it to adapt to the acid medium of the stomach is its ability to generate local alkali (ammonia) by splitting urea with its specific urease enzyme.

Epidemiology

H. pylori infection is worldwide but its mode of transmission is uncertain. Infection is more prevalent in lower socioeconomic groups and risk factors include poor living standards (such as crowded living conditions). In 'developed' westernised countries prevalence is low in children, but rises with increasing age, paralleling the age-related prevalence of chronic gastritis (20% of 20-year-olds and 60% of 60-year-olds). In poorer developing communities the prevalence is high in all age groups.

HELICOBACTER PYLORI INFECTIONS
Acute infection

There is little known about the acute phase of *H. pylori* infection. A short-lived illness with epigastric pain, nausea and vomiting associated with hypochlorhydria has been reported following ingestion of *H. pylori*. It is not known how frequently acute symptoms occur during the acquisition of *H. pylori* or what determines the outcome of acute infection. The consequences of chronic *H. pylori* infection are more important in clinical practice.

Chronic infection

H. pylori colonises epithelium of the gastric antrum in chronic infection (**57, 58**). The organism lies

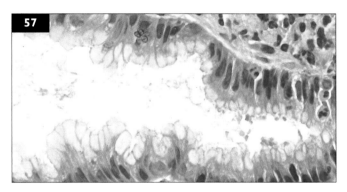

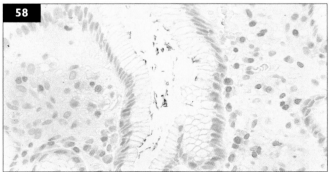

57 & 58 *Helicobacter pylori* seen at the surface of the gastric epithelium.

Helicobacter Pylori

adjacent to the gastric epithelial cells and in the gastric pits beneath the mucous layer. Active, chronic gastritis develops predominantly in the antrum. Degenerative changes occur in the epithelium and chronic inflammatory cells consisting of polymorphs, plasma cells and lymphocytes infiltrate the mucosa. Lymphoid aggregation and follicle formation also occurs in the basal mucosa.

These changes are not static and, over decades, progression from gastritis to atrophy to intestinal metaplasia probably occurs. The most severe gastritis is seen in young to middle-aged adults, whereas atrophic changes develop later in the disease process in older people. As gastric glands atrophy, the number of *H. pylori* falls as, paradoxically, this mucosa supports the organism less well. Finally, intestinal metaplasia develops with the presence of villiform structures and intestinal architecture. Advanced intestinal metaplasia is a factor in the development of gastric cancer.

Diagnosing *H. pylori* infection

Endoscopic methods There are no specific endoscopic features of *H. pylori* infection. Histological assessment of an endoscopic antral biopsy is a reliable means of detecting H. pylori, but is expensive, requires expertise, and the result is not immediately available. Culture of endoscopic biopsies is equally sensitive and specific but suffers similar drawbacks.

Several methods rely on the enzyme urease for *H. pylori* detection. Incubation of an infected antral biopsy in a solution of urea leads to the generation of ammonia by enzymatic degradation of urea. The subsequent pH change is visualised by a colour change in an indicator. Sensitivity is less than biopsy or culture, but these methods have the advantage of convenience, simplicity, and speed (a rapid version of this test can be read in 1 minute).

Breath tests The liberation of carbon dioxide in breath following urea ingestion can be used as a marker infection. When colonising the stomach break down labelled ingested urea to ammonia, carbon dioxide is released, absorbed, and excreted in the breath. Fasting subjects ingest isotopically labelled urea and a lipid drink (to impede gastric emptying) and after an interval breath is collected. This is analysed for the presence of labelled carbon dioxide. Use of either ^{13}C- or ^{14}C-labelled urea has been advocated. ^{13}C is a stable isotope, the advantage of which is that it is non-radioactive, but measurement requires a mass spectrometer.

^{14}C is radioactive, but it is detectable by the more widely available means of a scintillation counter. These tests are used to follow-up patients after attempts at eradication to determine whether or not this has been successful.

H. pylori serology Antibodies to detected by ELISA are indicative of current or past infection. Antibody titres fall after successful eradication of the organism. ELISA tests are being evaluated as a means of stratifying patients to determine those dyspeptic patients most likely to have organic disease (gastritis, peptic ulceration and cancer) at endoscopy.

DISEASE ASSOCIATIONS WITH *H. PYLORI*
Duodenal ulcer

There is a very strong association between chronic *H. pylori* infection and the development of duodenal ulceration. Up to 95% of patients with duodenal ulceration have evidence of *H. pylori* infection. However, it is important to recall that infection is very common in the general population.

Gastric ulceration

H. pylori infection is also strongly linked to the development of gastric ulcers, although not as closely as duodenal ulcers. Around 75–80% of gastric ulcer patients are infected.

Gastric cancer

The aetiology of gastric cancer is multifactorial and is incompletely understood.

It was appreciated before the current interest in *H. pylori* that gastric cancers often arose in areas of intestinal metaplasia and gastric atrophy. It has been suggested that *H. pylori* infection might facilitate the progression of changes from gastritis to gastric atrophy to intestinal metaplasia to gastric cancer. This hypothesis is based on the association between *H. pylori* infection rates shown by seroepidemiology and gastric cancer rates in different populations, and evidence of past *H. pylori* infection in patients with gastric cancer.

Mucosa-associated lymphoid tissue lymphomas (MALTomas)

MALTomas – B-cell lymphomas of the gastric mucosa – have been described in *H. pylori* infection. These are rare, low-grade lesions and there are reports of tumour regression on *H. pylori* eradication.

Helicobacter Pylori

Other associations

There are other associations with *H. pylori* infection, including the finding that *H. pylori*-infected children are smaller than their uninfected peers. An association with coronary heart disease has also been suggested.

'Non-ulcer dyspepsia' refers to the occurence of dyspeptic symptoms, without other upper GI pathology, in individuals with *H. pylori* infection. As the prevalence of *H. pylori* infection is high in the general population, the relevance of the association of the bacteria with such symptoms is uncertain.

TREATING *H. PYLORI* INFECTIONS

The ideal treatment for *H. pylori* would be simple, highly effective, lacking in side effects and cheap. This has proved difficult to achieve in practice, partly because of the ecological niche that *H. pylori* occupies, partly because of resistance to antibiotics, and partly because the acid pH of the stomach is far from optimal for antibiotic activity.

Eradication regimes are under constant review. Currently, antibiotic combinations, or combinations of antibiotics with acid suppression (e.g. proton pump inhibitor and clarithromycin or proton pump inhibitors and amoxycillin plus metronidazole or tinidazole) over different time scales all give high rates of eradication; this is defined as absent *H. pylori* 4 weeks after treatment has finished. Eradication rates reach 80–90%, providing that patient compliance with the multi-tablet regimes are good.

Eradication should be attempted in patients with ulcers as this reduces risk of duodenal ulcer recurrence. There is uncertainty over the benefits of eradication in patients with gastritis and, at the present time, no proven indication to eradicate patients with non-ulcer dyspepsia.

Chronic Gastric Ulcer

Definition
Chronic ulcers of the stomach are areas of mucosal ulceration extending to a variable (>1 mm) degree into the submucosal tissues. They can be complicated by perforation and haemorrhage.

Epidemiology
The life-time prevalence of gastric ulcer is 3% in females and 4% in males. Among the elderly, it may be more common in women. The median age at presentation is 50–60 years.

Pathophysiology
The pathogenesis of gastric ulceration is poorly understood. *H. pylori* is associated with 75–85% of gastric ulcers, a lower proportion than in duodenal ulceration. Also, basal and peak acid output is lower in patients with gastric ulcers than duodenal ulcer, probably because of the associated atrophic gastritis. Smoking is a risk factor.

Clinical history
Gastric ulcers can occur without symptoms. Symptomatic patients complain of attacks of epigastric pain lasting hours and often coming in cycles that last 6–8 weeks; the attacks may then abate for several months. Symptoms can be exacerbated by food. These complaints are non-specific and a variety of other upper gastrointestinal symptoms are reported, so that gastric ulcer cannot be differentiated from other causes of dyspepsia on clinical grounds.

Physical examination
Epigastric tenderness is found in some patients.

Laboratory and special examinations
Endoscopy and biopsy is the primary diagnostic modality (**59-61**). Barium studies continue to have a role (**62**). Gastric ulcers are found most frequently on the lesser curve at the junction of the antrum and body mucosa, as an oval or round lesion with slough-covered base. All gastric ulcers must be biopsied in each quadrant and floor to differentiate them from malignant ulcers. Concurrent endoscopic brushing for cytological assessment increases diagnostic accuracy. *H. pylori* should be sought, as this is more prevalent in gastric ulcer patients compared with controls.

Special forms
NSAIDs ulcers These drugs inhibit gastric prostaglandin synthesis and impair gastroduodenal mucosal defences and ulcer healing. Acute ingestion is associated with acute gastric erosions followed by an adaptive response over 1–2 months. Ulcers associated with chronic ingestion of NSAIDs are often asymptomatic until complicated by perforation or bleeding.

Resistant ulcers Ulcers failing to heal after 8 weeks' treatment with H_2 receptor antagonists are termed resistant. Biopsies should be repeated to be certain that the ulcer is not malignant. Surgery is indicated if the ulcer fails to heal after a further course of therapy.

Differential diagnosis
Between 4–10% of gastric ulcers are malignant, and so gastric cancer must be excluded in all gastric ulcers. Rolled irregular ulcer margins suggest malignancy (**63**) and ulcers >2 cm are four times more likely to be malignant than smaller ulcers. Endoscopy and biopsy must be repeated until the ulcer is healed.

Prognosis
Up to two-thirds of gastric ulcers will recur in 1 year.

MANAGEMENT OF GASTRIC ULCERS
General management
Smoking reduces ulcer healing and so should be discouraged. Diet makes no difference to healing rates.

Drugs
Acid suppression H_2 receptor antagonists have proved very successful in treating gastric ulcers. Healing rates are related to length of treatment and to the degree of 24-hour acid suppression, but after 8 weeks' treatment 80–90% of ulcers will be healed. There is little to choose between the different H_2 receptor antagonists.

Proton pump inhibitors are more potent at suppressing gastric acid and can also be used. Side effects limit the usefulness of anticholinergic drugs.

Mucosal protective agents Prostaglandins are important in regulating mucosal blood flow, re-epithelialisation after injury, and in mucus secretion. Misoprostil is a synthetic prostaglandin E_2 analogue that has mucosal protective and anti-secretory activity and is active in treating gastric ulcers.

Chronic Gastric Ulcer

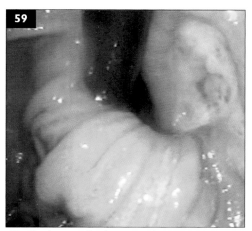

59 Benign gastric ulcer at endoscopy.

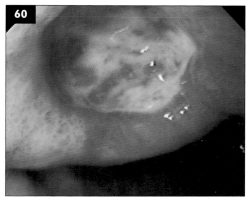

60 Benign gastric ulcer located at the incisura of the stomach.

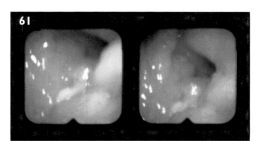

61 Small ulcer in pyloric channel seen at endoscopy.

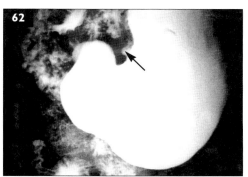

62 Barium meal showing benign gastric ulcer at incisura (arrowed).

Sucralfate, an aluminium salt of sucrose octasulphate, is a surface-acting agent that binds to the base of ulcers. It may also stimulate mucosal prostaglandins and can also used to treat gastric ulcers.

H. pylori eradication   *H. pylori* should be eradicated, although the importance of this in patients with gastric ulcer is less clear than in duodenal ulcer disease.

Maintenance H_2 receptor antagonist therapy As recurrent gastric ulceration is frequent and many recurrences are asymptomatic, patients often require maintenance H_2 receptor antagonist therapy. This is indicated for large (>2 cm) ulcers, those with a history of previous ulcers, patients who need to continue NSAIDs,

and elderly patients or those with concurrent cardiorespiratory disease that would make them particularly vulnerable in the event of an ulcer-related complication.

Surgery Indications for surgery are:
• Presence of complications (perforation, bleeding).
• Resistant ulcers.
• Suspicion of malignancy.
• Ulcers that relapse on maintenance therapy.
The usual operation is a Bilroth I partial gastrectomy, which reduces the parietal cell mass, but leaves the normal pathway of food from stomach to duodenum unchanged, although occasionally a Polya gastrectomy is performed (see section on 'Complications of Gastric Surgery', page 56, for a fuller description of these procedures).

Gastric Cancer

Definition
Primary cancer of the stomach.

Epidemiology
Gastric carcinoma is the most common cancer of the upper gastrointestinal tract. The incidence peaks between the ages of 55 and 65 years, and men are affected twice as often as women.

There are geographic variations in the disease prevalence, the cause of which is unknown. Chile and Japan, for instance, have especially high rates.

Aetiology
The aetiology of gastric cancer is multifactorial and a variety of factors have been implicated.

Dietary habits N-nitrosamine compounds are derived from dietary nitrates and nitrites by bacterial action and are directly carcinogenic. Diets rich in vitamins A, E and C are protective.

Environmental carcinogens These include alcohol and cigarette smoking.

Genetic factors Carriage of blood group A confers increased risk and there is a (minor) familial tendency. Risk is increased in patients with familial adenomatous polyposis.

H. pylori infection There is increasing evidence that acquisition of H. pylori at an early age is a risk factor in the development of gastric carcinoma. Chronic atrophic gastritis with intestinal metaplasia is recognised as a predisposing factor for gastric cancer and is also associated with infection. Both gastric cancer and are more prevalent in lower socioeconomic groups.

Adenomatous polyps These are uncommon, but have malignant potential.

Previous gastric surgery An increased incidence of gastric cancer is apparent 15–20 years after partial gastrectomy.

Patients with pernicious anaemia and achlorhydria have a small but increased risk.

Pathophysiology
Macroscopic appearances range from ulceration (**63**), to polypoid lesions, to diffuse infiltrative lesions (*linitis plastica*) (**64**). Ulcerative forms are most common, generally in the antrum and lesser curve. About 95% are adenocarcinomas and arise in areas of intestinal metaplasia.

The cancer may spread directly into adjacent structures or via the regional lymphatics which eventually drain into the cisterna chyli and thoracic duct. Peritoneal spread is common and ovarian deposits (Krukenberg tumours) may occur.

Clinical history
Symptoms are often vague in the early stages. There are no features to distinguish dyspepsia associated with gastric cancer from benign causes, but the history is usually short (<1 year). Anorexia and weight loss is frequent as disease advances. Haematemesis occurs, but is unusual. Early satiety may be a prominent feature of diffuse infiltrating carcinoma (*linitis plastica*) due to immobility of the stomach wall. Gastric outlet obstruction may be a late feature of advanced antral carcinoma, with nausea and vomiting.

Physical examination
In patients with disease confined to the stomach there are no physical signs, but 25% of patients present with metastatic disease in the lungs, liver, bone and brain. Evidence of metastases may be detected clinically – including Troisier's sign, involvement of the left supraclavicular nodes. Non-metastatic manifestations include acanthosis nigricans, thrombophlebitis migrans (Trousseau's sign) and dermatomyositis.

Laboratory and special investigations
Diagnosis is usually suspected at gastroscopy, and endoscopic biopsy is always indicated following radiological diagnosis of gastric ulcer. Multiple biopsies and brushing are required from each quadrant of the ulcer to ensure the diagnosis is not missed. Radiography, CT, ultrasound and bone scan are used to detect metastatic disease when this is appropriate.

Special forms
'Early' gastric cancer is a term used to denote gastric cancer that is curable and recognisable endoscopically, although endoscopic changes may be very subtle. Lesions are confined to the mucosa but, paradoxically, may have venous metastases. In Japan, 5-year survival rates of 90% have been reported using limited barium meal or endoscopy in mass screening programmes to detect early gastric cancer.

Gastric Cancer

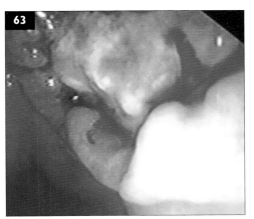

63 A classical rolled edge of a malignant gastric ulcer.

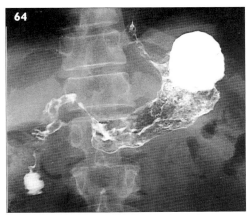

64 Gastric cancer of the 'Linitis plastica' type – this constricted stomach wall is diffusely infiltrated and the stomach cannot dilate.

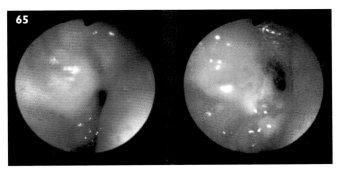

65 Recurrent gastric cancer after resection.

Differential diagnosis
As the symptoms of gastric cancer in the early, curable, stage are non-specific, it is imperative that the diagnosis is considered in all patients aged over 40 and presenting with dyspepsia. Equally, since benign and malignant gastric ulcers can have identical macroscopic appearances, all gastric ulcers must be biopsied repeatedly in different sites and followed up endoscopically until healed in order to avoid misdiagnosis.

Prognosis
Overall, the 5-year survival rate is 10%, and for inoperable disease the mean interval from diagnosis to death is 4 months (**65**). Histological tumour grade and spread are prognostic.

Management
Surgery This offers the only potentially curative treatment in selected patients. Curative surgery includes excision of the tumour, omentum and lymphatics draining the area. Surgical palliation should be considered for obstruction, haemorrhage and pain.

Adjuvant chemotherapy This has little to offer, although recently there has been interest in the use of 5-fluorouracil and cisplatin.

Other treatments Dyspeptic symptoms may respond to acid suppression, but opiates are usually required for pain eventually. Liaison with family, the family practitioner and palliative care specialist is important in the terminal stages.

Complications of Gastric Surgery

Gastric surgery (**66**) was once commonplace, but with the decline in peptic ulcer disease and newer pharmacological approaches to its management and the recognition of the value of *H. pylori* eradication in preventing ulcer recurrence, this has changed.

Similar complications are shared by all types of gastric surgery, but their respective frequency varies with different operations. Most patients get some symptoms but, in general, they improve during the first 6–12 months after surgery.

STOMACH, MARGINAL OR ANASTOMOTIC ULCERS

Ulceration may occur at anastomotic sites where acid-producing gastric mucosa is directly adjacent to duodenal or small intestinal mucosa (**67**). Symptoms are similar to those of any peptic ulcer. Acid reduction by H_2 antagonists or proton pump inhibitors will help, but re-operation may be necessary to further reduce acide production.

EARLY DUMPING

Rapid emptying of gastric contents into the small bowel causes symptoms of abdominal pain, diarrhoea, nausea and systemic symptoms of faintness, sweating and palpitations within 30 minutes of eating. Three mechanisms are proposed.
- Intestinal distension may initiate autonomic reflexes that cause symptoms.
- Hyperosmolar stomach contents lead to a swift osmotic transfer of fluid out of the vascular compartment into the gut lumen, and transient hypovolaemia.
- Release of gastrointestinal hormones.

Early dumping is managed by advising small, low-carbohydrate meals taken frequently with liquid. Guar may reduce symptoms. Further surgical intervention is reserved for intractable symptoms persisting for more than a year after operation.

Paradoxically, gastric stasis can also be a sequel to gastric surgery. This is usually because of impaired drainage following vagotomy. The procedure of truncal vagotomy to reduce acid was always accompanied by a gastric drainage procedure (pyloroplasty or gastroenterostomy) to aid drainage.

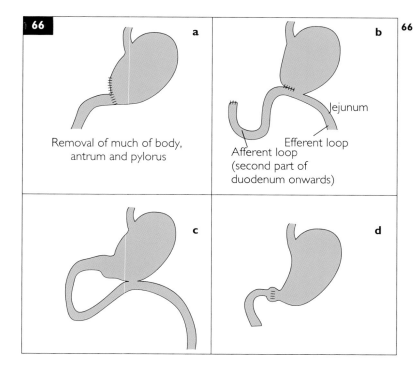

66 Diagram of main gastric operations. (a) Bilroth I partial gastrectomy. (b) Polya or Bilroth II partial gastrectomy. (c) Gastrojejunostomy. (d) Pyloroplasty. For benign disease, operations would either reduce the amount of acid-secreting mucosa (a,b), or drain the stomach after vagotomy (c,d) (as cutting the vagus to reduce acid results in a non-functioning pylorus).

66

a Removal of much of body, antrum and pylorus

b Jejunum / Efferent loop / Afferent loop (second part of duodenum onwards)

c

d

Complications of Gastric Surgery

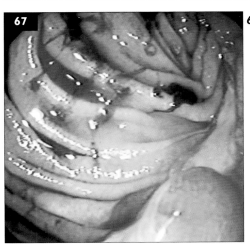

67 A stomal ulcer seen at endoscopy. The patient has had a Polya gastrectomy with afferent and efferent loops and the ulcer is at the margin of the gastric and small intestinal mucosa.

LATE DUMPING

Rapid absorption of carbohydrate may cause an inappropriate release of insulin from the pancreas, and faintness and dizziness due to reactive hypoglycaemia 1–2 hours after eating. Treatment is similar to that for early dumping.

DIARRHOEA

This may occur due to changes in motility and rapid fluid transfer through the small intestine and colon.

Symptoms occur within 1–2 hours of eating. Treatment is as for early dumping. Some patients benefit from anti-diarrhoeal agents or bile salt binding with cholestyramine.

BILIOUS VOMITING

Loss of the antropyloric barrier may allow reflux of duodenal contents into the stomach. Bile and pancreatic enzymes are irritant and cause gastritis.

The endoscopic appearance has been termed the 'red and green' stomach – friable erythematous mucosa with green bilious fluid. Patients complain of pain, and may vomit bile-stained fluid. The management includes bile acid-binding agents (e.g. cholestyramine) and prokinetic agents (e.g. cisapride). Reflux gastropathy is independent of the post-surgical gastritis and stomal ulceration (**67**) seen commonly at endoscopy in post-surgical stomachs.

GASTRO-OESOPHAGEAL REFLUX

Lower oesophageal sphincter tone is reduced after gastric surgery, both directly due to vagotomy and due to loss of normal reflex and hormonal responses to eating. Bile reflux may also contribute.

CANCER IN THE REMNANT STOMACH

The absolute risk and mechanism is debated, but following gastric surgery the risk of gastric cancer is increased.

METABOLIC COMPLICATIONS AFTER GASTRIC SURGERY
Anaemia

Iron-deficiency is common due to stomal ulceration, post-surgical gastritis and reduced iron absorption. Megaloblastic anaemia due to B_{12} deficiency, as a result of reduction in intrinsic factor and therefore ileal malabsorption of B_{12}, may occur after a delay of many years.

Osteomalacia

This is also more common from calcium and vitamin D deficiency.

Weight loss

Weight loss after surgery is almost inevitable. It occurs because of inadequate food intake (partly because of dietary changes necessitated by dumping and diarrhoea), and malabsorption. The cause of malabsorption is not well understood, but mild degrees of steatorrhoea are common. Both bacterial overgrowth and disordered motility may contribute.

Disorders of Gastric Motility and Bezoars

Definition
The normal stomach has rhythmic contractions that both control and propel the boluses of food entering the small intestine. This is disturbed in a number of disease states.

Epidemiology and aetiology
See 'Special forms' below.

Pathophysiology
As food enters the stomach, the gastric fundus relaxes to accommodate it, after which peristaltic waves push it down to the antrum. The peristaltic process is mediated by vagal reflexes and the local intrinsic gastric plexuses.

Vagotomy or partial gastrectomy impairs accommodation, resulting in inability to consume large meals, and leads to rapid gastric emptying.

Impaired emptying results from deregulated or disordered peristalsis, and leads to delayed gastric emptying.

Disordered peristalsis may underlie the development of gastric diverticulae (**68**).

Clinical history
Impaired accommodation Patients complain of early satiety and postprandial fullness.

Rapid early emptying This gives rise to 'dumping' and postprandial diarrhoea, and is seen as a complication of gastric surgery.

Delayed gastric emptying Patients experience upper abdominal pain, fullness, nausea and vomiting. The vomiting can be projectile, and food ingested many hours or even several days previously may be seen in the vomitus. Delayed gastric emptying may occur due to conditions distorting anatomy (e.g. pyloric stenosis, antral cancer) or because of a disorder affecting neural function (e.g. diabetes). In some of the latter, the cause is unknown.

Physical examination
In those with delayed gastric emptying, there may be evidence of weight loss, the dilated stomach can be palpable, and there is sometimes a succussion splash (audible splash over stomach on shaking the abdomen).

Laboratory and special examinations
Barium radiology will detect food debris in the stomach and give an estimate of emptying, but scintigraphic measures of gastric emptying following a standard meal with a radiolabelled tracer offer the most sensitive test. Endoscopy is usually required to exclude mechanical obstruction, ideally after nasogastric drainage of gastric contents. Aspiration of >150 ml of fluid from the stomach after an overnight fast is suggestive of delayed gastric emptying.

Special forms and complications
Bezoars Stasis predisposes to gastric bezoars – aggregates of indigestible material which form residue trapped in the antrum. Phytobezoars are made of concretions of fibrous vegetable material, but bezoars made of a number of other materials have been described. Trichobezoars are made of hair and food debris and are most common in young women who habitually eat hair, but some patients are psychiatrically disturbed (**69**).

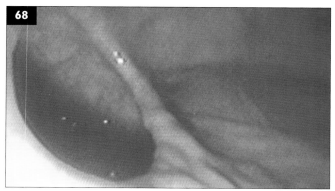

68 A diverticulum in the fundus of the stomach.

Disorders of Gastric Motility and Bezoars

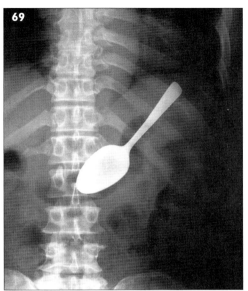

69 Ingested foreign body, lying within the gas pattern of the gastric outline.

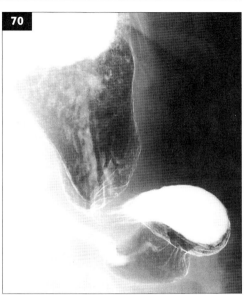

70 Gastric volvulus. Note the rotation of the stomach around its long axis.

Patients present with pain, nausea and fullness. The bezoar may be palpable, and can be confirmed by barium meal or endoscopy. Complications include gastritis, ulceration and anaemia.

Management consists of endoscopic disintegration of the bezoar and treating the impaired motility.

Diabetic gastroparesis Gastroparesis is a manifestation of diabetic autonomic neuropathy involving the vagal nerve and intrinsic plexuses of the stomach. The typical symptoms are delayed gastric emptying and, because food is delivered erratically to the duodenum, poor diabetic control. Often symptoms vary from week to week. Treatment consists of optimising diabetic control, and use of prokinetic agents. Erythromycin – a motilin agonist – has also been advocated.

Gastric volvulus (**70**) In individuals with long, thin stomachs, rotation around the long axis of the stomach may occur. This presents with severe pain, and vomiting with only low volumes of vomitus. It often settles spontaneously, but surgical intervention may be needed.

Differential diagnosis

Mechanical obstruction of the gastric outlet causes delayed gastric emptying (see **68**). In adults, this is most commonly due to pyloric stenosis by peptic ulcer disease or carcinoma. Adult hypertrophic pyloric stenosis is rare.

Delayed gastric emptying can be due to drugs such as opiates, and drugs with anticholinergic effects like tricyclic antidepressants.

It is also common in patients with gastro-oesophageal reflux and up to 50% of patients with non-ulcer dyspepsia have delayed gastric emptying, but the relationship of this to symptoms is unclear.

Dermatomyositis, scleroderma and myotonic muscular dystrophy are also causes of abnormal gastric motility.

Prognosis

The prognosis depends on the cause. It is poor in diabetic gastroparesis, since it usually occurs in association with autonomic neuropathy and other complications of long-standing diabetes.

Management

Prokinetic drugs such as metoclopramide, domperidone and cisapride should be tried.

Ménétrier's Disease and Other Rugal Hyperplastic Gastropathies

Definition
The rugal hyperplastic gastropathies are a group of poorly understood diseases in which giant gastric folds (rugae) are found at endoscopy or on radiological evaluation.

Epidemiology and aetiology
Ménétrier's disease This is a rare condition that may occur at any age and affects men more than women. The aetiology is unknown, although the growth factor TGF-alpha is prominent in the gastric tissue.

Zollinger–Ellison syndrome This is a rare, sporadic or genetic condition in which rugal hypertrophy occurs as a response to excess production of the hormone gastrin by a neuroendocrine tumour, often located in the pancreas or duodenum (page 45).

Hypertrophic hypersecretory gastritis A rare condition with giant folds, high acid excretion, but not associated with neuroendocrine tumours.

Ménétrier's pathophysiology
The characteristic macroscopic feature is mucus-covered giant cerebriform rugae, especially in the fundus (71, 72). There may be haemorrhage and erosions associated with areas of rugal hypertrophy. The key histological feature is mucous cell hyperplasia, and cystic dilatation of gastric glands submucosally. Gastric acidity is reduced as a consequence of gland atrophy and excess mucus, and protein loss occurs from the stomach.

Clinical history
The patient may give a history of indigestion.

Physical examination
There is peripheral oedema and, in severe protein loss, ascites may be present.

Laboratory and special investigations
The diagnosis is suggested by finding enlarged tortuous rugae in the corpus and greater curve of the stomach. Large endoscopic biopsies are required to examine the gland architecture. Blood investigations may reveal hypoproteinaemia. Protein loss can be documented by retrieval of labelled albumin from gastric aspirates, but is rarely performed.

Differential diagnosis
Ménétrier's disease is differentiated from gastric carcinoma and lymphoma by endoscopic biopsy and endoscopic ultrasound. Giant rugae are also a feature of hypertrophic hypersecretory gastropathy, but this is associated with increased gastric acid secretion and normogastrinaemia. In Zollinger–Ellison syndrome, there is rugal hypertrophy, hypergastrinaemia causing parietal cell hyperplasia and consequent excess acid that leads to peptic ulceration and diarrhoea.

Prognosis
Ménétrier's disease usually runs a protracted course.

Management
There is no specific therapy for Ménétrier's disease. Acid suppression with H_2 receptor antagonists, proton pump inhibitors or anticholinergic drugs have been tried. Surgery is reserved for patients with persistent hypoproteinaemia, blood loss and refractory symptoms. For hypertrophic hypersecretory gastritis and Zollinger–Ellison syndrome, acid suppression is the mainstay of the treatment.

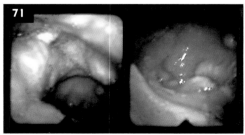

71 Endoscopic appearances of Ménétrier's disease with oedematous gastric folds.

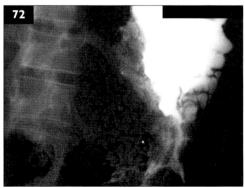

72 Giant gastric folds seen on barium meal in Ménétrier's disease (source of protein loss).

Gastric Antral Vascular Ectasia (Synonym Watermelon Stomach)

Definition
Diffuse vascular ectasia of the stomach antrum.

Epidemiology and aetiology
This condition is more common in females (typically, a female:male ratio of 8:1). In some patients, there is an association with cirrhosis, and with reduced serum gastrin levels.

Pathophysiology
The lesions are dilated ectatic vessels surrounded by fibrosis. In cirrhosis they may develop from intramural vascular shunts caused by portal hypertension.

Clinical history
Patients present with overt or covert gastro-intestinal bleeding.

Physical examination
There may be evidence of anaemia and signs of cirrhosis.

Laboratory and special investigations
The diagnosis is usually made at endoscopy. Typically, red/blue lesions are clustered on the crests of longitudinal rugal folds that converge on the pylorus, like stripes on a watermelon. Scattered rounded lesions are also seen.

The lesions are strings of telangiectatic vessels that blanch on pressure of biopsy forceps, and bleed excessively if biopsied (**73**).

Prognosis
The lesions continue to bleed intermittently and chronically in most patients.

Management
A variety of approaches has been tried. Antrectomy is the most radical. Endoscopic therapies include alcohol injection and laser ablation. Corticosteroids and oestrogen–progesterone have also been used. Patients need endoscopic follow-up as ablated lesions tend to return.

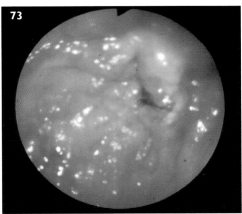

73 'Haemorrhagic' streaks of gastric vascular ectasia.

Gastric Polyps and Benign Gastric Tumours

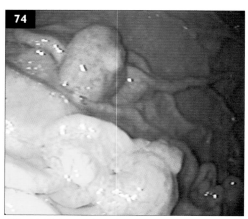

74 Multiple gastric polyps seen at endoscopy.

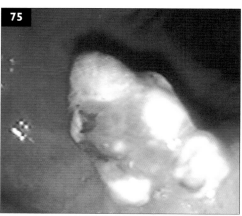

75 A gastric adenoma at the oesophagogastric junction. The histology was surprisingly benign.

Definition
'Gastric polyp' is a generic term that describes a variety of pathologies causing polypoid lesions in the stomach. They must be differentiated histologically.

Epidemiology
Patients usually present in the sixth and seventh decades; males and females are equally affected. Although post mortem studies suggest gastric polyps are uncommon, they are found in 1–3% of the (selected) population that undergo endoscopy.

Pathophysiology: epithelial lesions
Benign gastric epithelial lesions are important because they are all, to varying degrees, pre-malignant and potentially curable endoscopically. The aetiology is unknown, but they occur in atrophic mucosa, often in association with intestinal metaplasia and are more frequent in achlorhydric patients.

Hyperplastic polyps (regenerative polyps) These are the most common gastric polyps and account for two-thirds of lesions. They usually occur in the gastric fundus and body as multiple sessile lesions (**74**) and have limited if any malignant potential. They are an overgrowth of gastric foveolar and gland tissue. Multiple biopsies are often needed to differentiate them from adenomatous polyps.

Benign adenomatous gastric polyps Benign adenomatous gastric polyps arise from gastric glands and tend to occur predominantly in the antrum. Usually they are solitary, pedunculated and have tubulovillous architecture (**75**). There is a significant risk of malignant change, especially in lesions >2 cm in size.

Pathophysiology: non-epithelial lesions
Non-epithelial lesions are much less common and, because they are predominantly submucosal, more difficult to diagnose endoscopically.

Leiomyomas Leiomyomas arise in the smooth muscle layers and expand submucosally towards the lumen (**76**). Their apex may ulcerate the mucosa, and lead to presentation with haematemesis. Some also involve the serosal surface of the stomach – 'dumb-bell' tumours. Malignant transformation to leiomyosarcoma may occur.

Other non-epithelial tumours Submucosal lipomas can be recognised, as they are compressible at endoscopy. Neurogenic and vascular tumours also occur.
Ectopic pancreatic tissue can also occur in the antrum and present as an intramucosal lesion. Very rarely, intramural gastric duplication cysts cause a smooth indentation in the stomach wall.

Clinical history
There are no specific symptoms. Patients present with dyspepsia, nausea or weight loss. Anaemia is common, but frank haematemesis rare.

Gastric Polyps and Benign Gastric Tumours

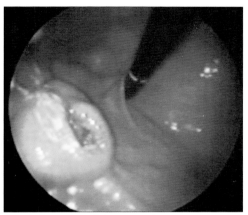

76 Leiomyoma of the stomach.

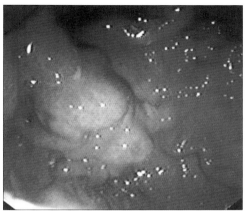

77 Not a tumour, but a fundal varix in the presence of portal hypertension.

Intermittent gastric outlet obstruction can occur with pedunculated antral lesions.

Physical examination
This is usually normal.

Laboratory and special examinations
Endoscopic excision of the whole polyp offers the most certain means of diagnosis. Not all 'polypoid' lesions seen in the stomach are true polyps, and prominent normal folding can be mistaken for a polyp. Patients with polyps seen on barium meal must be referred for endoscopy. Parietal cell and intrinsic factor antibodies, and vitamin B_{12} estimation are indicated to detect pernicious anaemia in patients with adenomas. The large bowel should also be investigated as there is an association with colonic polyps.

The diagnosis of non-epithelial lesions is problematic: endoscopic biopsy may not be adequate for diagnosis in submucosal lesions and the behaviour of leiomyomas – the most common submucosal lesion – is difficult to predict. Endoscopic ultrasound has proved valuable in diagnosis and for differentiating submucosal lesions from extra-gastric compression.

CT scanning may show the characteristic low attenuation appearances of lipomas.

Special forms
Several polyposis syndromes are recognised. Adenomatous polyps are found in the stomach and duodenum of patients with familial adenomatous polyposis. The polyps in patients with Peutz–Jehger's syndrome are hamartoma with little malignant potential, but warrant endoscopic removal to reduce the risk of intusussception. In Cronkhite–Canada syndrome (hyperpigmentation, alopecia, nail dystrophy and polyposis) polyps are similar to those in Ménétrier's disease.

Differential diagnosis
Extrinsic compression of the stomach may mimic submucosal tumours or ectopic pancreatic tissue. Gastric lymphoma can be polypoid, and polypoid swelling of rugae occurs in Ménétrier's disease. Carcinoid and amyloid are rare causes of polypoid lesions. Gastric varices due to portal hypertension may appear polypoid (**77**) and should not be biopsied!

Prognosis
Generally good, unless malignant change occurs.

Management
The management depends on the histology of the polyp. Small pedunculated polyps can be excised endoscopically and patients followed up with endoscopic surveillance. In the frail and elderly, this is preferable to surgery and its attendant risks. Patients with rapidly recurring or neoplastic polyps should be offered surgery.

Gastric Lymphoma

Definition
Primary gastrointestinal lymphoma of the stomach.

Epidemiology and aetiology
Primary lymphomas of the gastrointestinal tract are rare, but the stomach is the most common site, accounting for about half of all primary gastrointestinal lymphomas (**78**).

Peak incidence occurs in the 60-year-old age group, with men affected more frequently than women.

Pathophysiology
Gastric lymphomas present as an ulcer, a diffuse infiltrating lesion or with giant rugal folds mimicking Ménétrier's disease. Most gastric lymphomas are B-cell lymphomas. Recently, an association between low-grade lymphoma and *H. pylori* has been recognised, and there are reports of regression of the these low-grade tumours, limited to the mucosa, following eradication of *H. pylori*, suggesting that in some cases at least the aberrant lymphocyte proliferation is driven by the presence of the bacterium.

Clinical history
Non-specific dyspepsia, anorexia, weight loss, nausea and vomiting.

Physical examination
An epigastric mass is palpable in 30% of patients.

Laboratory and special investigations
There is commonly anaemia and raised ESR. Endoscopic appearances of lymphomatous lesions are similar to those of gastric cancer, but diagnosis is frequently delayed as biopsies are often falsely negative since the lymphomatous tissue is deep in the mucosa. Multiple snare biopsies are more likely to yield the diagnosis. Radiologically, extension of a lesion from stomach into duodenum is suggestive of gastric lymphoma.

Bone marrow examination and thoraco-abdominal imaging are necessary to differentiate from other extranodal lymphomas.

Differential diagnosis
Gastric lymphoma is frequently misdiagnosed as gastric ulcer. The true diagnosis emerges when the lesion fails to heal. Some are only diagnosed by frozen section from exploratory laparotomy. Primary gastric lymphoma can generally be differentiated from a secondary lymphoma spreading from other sites by: the absence of palpable lymphadenopathy, no mediastinal lymphadenopathy, and only regional/retroperitoneal lymph node involvement, no hepatic or splenic involvement other than by direct spread, normal bone marrow, and disease confined mainly to the gastrointestinal tract. These criteria no longer pertain in very advanced cases.

Prognosis
The prognosis is better than that for gastric cancer, and 5-year survival rates can exceed 75%. Features associated with good prognosis include; early stage disease, small (<10 cm) size, diffuse histiocytic or large cell histological types, and a good initial response.

Management
Conventionally, lesions confined to the stomach are treated surgically and radiotherapy and chemotherapy are used in advanced disease.

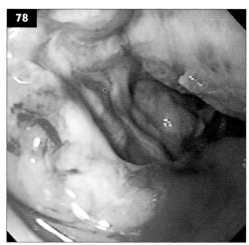

78 Gastro-duodenal lymphoma.

Duodenum: Anatomy and Histology

The duodenum passes from the pylorus to the duodenojejunal flexure – a distance of about 30 cm in a normal adult (**79**). There are four parts: the first (the 'duodenal bulb') is 3–5 cm long and is the prime site for duodenal ulcers; the second is 7–10 cm long and receives biliary and pancreatic drainage via the ampulla of Vater; the third and fourth parts complete the duodenal 'loop'. From the ligament of Treitz onwards, the upper small intestine is named the jejunum.

Histology

The histology of the duodenal mucosa is similar to that of the other small intestine regions. The intestinal surface of the mucosa and submucosa is thrown into multiple villi, which increase the absorptive area. Specialised epithelial cells are absorptive, with further specialised microvilli on the surface. A unique feature of the duodenum is the presence of Brunner's glands in the submucosal layer (**80**).

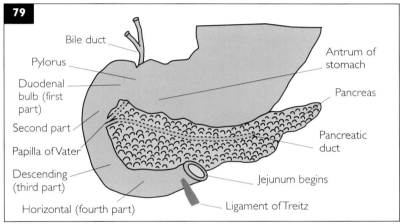

79 Anatomy of the duodenum.

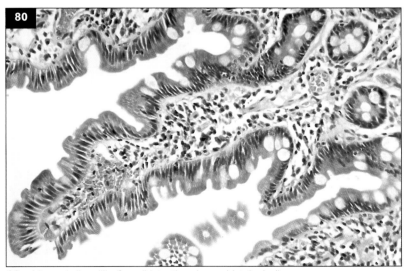

80 Normal slim villi of small intestine shown histologically.

Chronic Duodenal Ulceration

Definition
Chronic ulceration of the duodenum is a common clinical problem and describes the presence of a breach in the duodenal mucosa that has depth. Duodenitis shares a similar aetiology and refers to inflammation in the duodenum. Endoscopically, duodenitis is associated with erosions which are smaller superficial lesions of the mucosa – an appearance called 'salt and pepper duodenitis'.

Epidemiology
Duodenal ulcers are common in all age groups, but incidence rises with age (c.f. gastric ulcers which are rare below 40 years). The lifetime prevalence of duodenal ulceration is about 10% for men and 4% for women, but duodenal ulcer prevalence is falling.

Pathophysiology
H. pylori is the most important acquired factor in aetiology and over 95% of duodenal ulcer patients are infected. The mechanism whereby antral infection with *H. pylori* results in ulceration in the duodenum is conjectural. Gastric acid and pepsin are important, and both basal and stimulated gastric acid secretion are higher in duodenal ulcer patients secondary to hypergastrinaemia. This may be attributable to *H. pylori* infection as may the apparent familial clustering of duodenal ulcer disease. Alternatively, familial clustering could be linked directly to heritable factors; for instance, blood group O non-secretor status confers risk. Other factors include cirrhosis and chronic pancreatitis, smoking and low socioeconomic class.

Clinical history
Patients complain of dyspepsia in relation to food – worsening the pain in some and relieving symptoms in others. Patients complain of many other upper gastrointestinal symptoms and, as with gastric ulcers, these are non-discriminatory.

Physical examination
Usually, the physical examination is normal. Epigastric tenderness can sometimes be elicited.

Laboratory and special examinations
Barium meal radiology will detect most duodenal ulcers (**81**, **82**) and is better than endoscopy for examining the distal duodenum. Endoscopy is more sensitive, can distinguish active ulceration from previous scarring, and can detect very small mucosal lesions (**83**). Antral biopsies can also be taken to diagnose *H. pylori* at the time of endoscopy.

Special forms
Zollinger–Ellison syndrome patients develop multiple duodenal ulcers secondary to gastrin secretion by tumour. Ulcers can involve the distal duodenum (which is unusual in straightforward peptic ulceration) and some patients have diarrhoea.

Differential diagnosis
Rarely, duodenal ulceration is a manifestation of Crohn's disease, tuberculosis, lymphoma or sarcoidosis and, in immunocompromised patients, cytomegalovirus. (In practice an *H. pylori*-negative duodenal ulcer and lesions distal to the first part of the duodenum should alert the endoscopist to the possibility of these diagnoses.) Pancreatic cancers can erode into the duodenum. Duodenal cancer is very rare.

Prognosis
The natural history of duodenal ulcer disease is relapsing and remitting unless *H. pylori* is eradicated. Without such eradication, about 80% of patients relapse within a year of healing. Ulcer perforation and bleeding are the most important complications, and chronic duodenal ulceration can lead to pyloric stenosis.

Management
General management Smoking impairs ulcer healing and increases relapse, so it should be discouraged. NSAIDs should be discontinued if feasible.

Acid suppression Duodenal ulcers heal faster than gastric ulcers because they are smaller and H_2 receptor antagonists will rapidly heal 90% of duodenal ulcers in 6 weeks. Proton pump inhibitors heal even faster. Resistant ulcers are usually due to smoking, poor compliance, or both.

Maintenance H_2 receptor antagonist therapy Indications for maintenance H_2 receptor antagonist therapy include: elderly patients (or those with concurrent cardiorespiratory disease), smokers, previous ulcer complication, frequent relapses, severe/protracted symptoms during relapse and co-prescription of NSAIDs in patients with known or previous ulceration. Half the healing dose is given during maintenance. Alternative approaches to preventing ulcer disease with NSAIDs include the simultaneous use of prostaglandin analogues.

Chronic Duodenal Ulceration

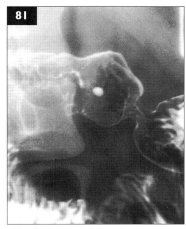

81 Barium meal showing an acute duodenal ulcer as a small round pool of barium.

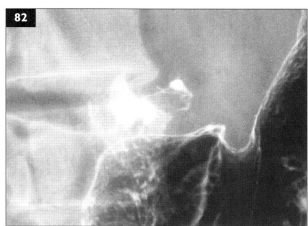

82 A chronic deformed duodenal cap due to long-standing duodenal ulceration, seen on barium meal.

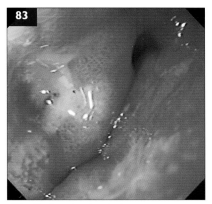

83 Kissing duodenal ulcers.

H. pylori eradication Indications for eradication of *H. pylori* are continually being reviewed. All infected ulcer patients are now thought to require *H. pylori* eradication, though previously this was advised only in recurrent/complicated ulcers. Eradication of *H. pylori* reduces the relapse rate to <10% per year. It is likely that the long-term complications of bleeding and perforation will show a similar trend.

Surgery Surgery is indicated for complications and severe and refractory duodenal ulceration. The highly selective vagotomy is the procedure of choice, as gastric emptying is unimpaired. Former operations included vagotomy and pyloroplasty, vagotomy and gastroenterostomy, and partial gastrectomy (Bilroth II). With the advent of more potent acid suppression and the recognition and eradication of *H. pylori* infection, surgery for duodenal ulceration is becoming less frequent.

Complications of Peptic Ulcers

The most important complications of peptic ulceration (both gastric and duodenal) are gastrointestinal bleeding and perforation. With duodenal ulcers and antropyloric ulceration there is also the long-term complication of pyloric stenosis due to scarring and distortion of the pylorus from chronic and recurrent inflammation.

PERFORATION

Typically, patients present with severe sudden abdominal pain, and lie still with a rigid abdomen, pale, hypotensive, and very ill. A plain chest radiograph will generally reveal air under the diaphragm (**84**). Perforated peptic ulcer is a surgical emergency. There are reports of conservative management of perforated duodenal ulcers in younger patients: as yet, this is not routine and laparotomy is currently the accepted approach.

The operative management of perforated duodenal ulcer is either simple closure or a definitive procedure to decrease gastric acidity. The experience of the surgeon, the condition of the patient, and the presence of established peritonitis are all factors. Definitive surgery involves closure of the perforation, drainage and either truncal or highly selective vagotomy.

Perforated gastric ulcers are usually excised at operation because of the risk of malignancy, and reoperation is more frequently required after oversewing a perforated gastric ulcer than duodenal ulcer. The prognosis is worse as patients are older and the peritonitis is more severe.

BLEEDING PEPTIC ULCERS

Bleeding peptic ulcers account for about 50% of acute upper gastrointestinal haemorrhage in the UK. With NSAID and aspirin use, there is a four-fold increased risk of bleeding. Diagnosis is best made by early endoscopy (**85**).

Management

The patient should be resuscitated with blood and colloid.

Pharmacological therapy This has been disappointing, and no convincing benefit has been demonstrated to accrue from acid suppression or anti-fibrinolytic therapy.

Endoscopic treatment Endoscopic interventions to arrest bleeding from ulcers are becoming commonplace. Application of endoscopic heater probes, laser coagulation, electrocoagulation and injection sclerotherapy have all been tried. The best

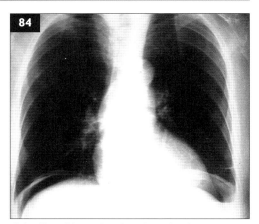

84 Chest X-ray showing 'air under the diaphragm' or pneumoperitoneum – following perforation of duodenal ulcer.

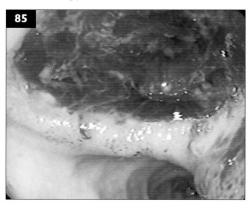

85 Duodenal ulcer with clot in base.

approach is not yet known. Actively bleeding ulcers or those with evidence of recent bleeding (for example a black spot in the base) should receive interventional treatments at endoscopy.

Surgery Normally, 90% of bleeding ulcers stop bleeding with conservative management. The indications for surgery and its timing are controversial. Patients are most successfully managed when there is close liaison between the surgeons and physicians. There should be a low threshold for surgery in an elderly patient with coexistent illness, and a higher threshold for previously fit young patients.

The operation of choice for bleeding duodenal ulcer is vagotomy and pyloroplasty. Gastric ulcers are managed by Billroth I gastrectomy.

Chapter Five

Jejunum and Ileum

The diseases predominantly affecting the jejunum and ileum are inflammatory, and tumours are relatively uncommon

Investigation of malabsorption is a pragmatic exercise, based on identifying evidence for malabsorption from blood tests, and securing an anatomical explanation by radiology and biopsy

Immunodeficiency can present with small intestinal infections

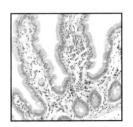
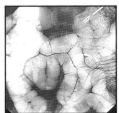
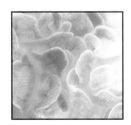
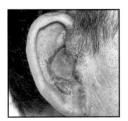

Anatomy and Histology

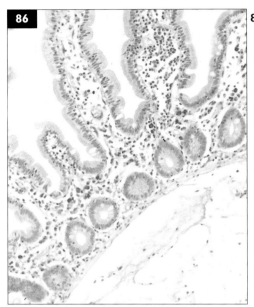

86 Histological appearance of normal villi of the small intestine.

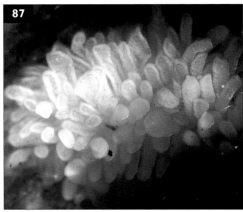

87 Normal dissecting microscope appearances of finger-like villi.

In the normal adult, the small intestine is about 6 metres in length. The change from the jejunum to the ileum occurs at about the half-way point. The jejunum is predominantly in the left upper quadrant; the ileum predominantly in the right lower quadrant, unless malrotation has occurred during foetal development. In about 2% of people, at about 60 cm (2 ft) from the ileocaecal valve, is Meckel's diverticulum, a residuum of the developmental umbilical tract, located on the opposite side from that on which the mesentery is attached (antimesenteric border). Meckel's diverticulum is usually 5–8 cm long and may contain ectopic gastric mucosa.

Microscopically, the jejunum and ileum, like the duodenum, demonstrate multiple villi, finger-like protrusions of the mucosa, which increase the absorptive area (**86, 87**).

Investigations of the Small Intestine

SMALL-BOWEL RADIOLOGY
This may be used to demonstrate anatomy. There are two techniques:
- Barium follow-through – ingestion of barium. Small-bowel radiographs are taken as the barium moves spontaneously through the intestine (**88**). This is a slow procedure.
- Small-bowel enema: this involves naso-duodenal or jejunal intubation (under fluoroscopy) followed by rapid infusion of liquid barium (**89**). While preferred by some radiologists, patients often find this a difficult procedure.

The appearances of the two techniques differ. In disease, they may show dilatation of the bowel, thickening of bowel wall, strictures, fistulas and tumours. A technical problem may occur due to barium flocculating in the presence of malabsorption.

OTHER TESTS
Jejunal biopsy
This is performed using a pneumatic capsule, e.g. Crosby capsule, under fluoroscopy. The method provides a representative sample of mucosa, so that dissecting microscope appearances can be visualised (**90**). On the whole, this has been replaced by duodenal biopsy at endoscopy (**91**) for identification of diffuse small-intestinal disease (e.g. coeliac disease).

Investigations of the Small Intestine

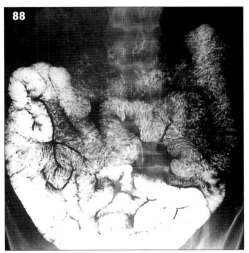

88 Classical small bowel follow-through appearance, again with jejunum at upper left and ileum at lower right.

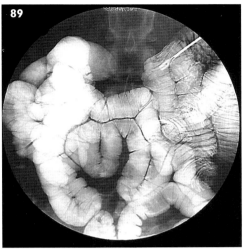

89 Normal appearances of intubated small bowel enema, demonstrating jejunum on upper right and ileum on lower left.

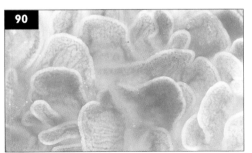

90 Broad, leafy villi with some finger-like villi, in a patient with scleroderma.

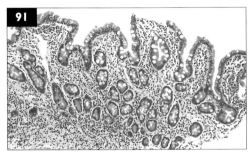

91 Partial villous atrophy in a patient with coeliac disease recovering on a gluten-free diet.

Small-intestinal endoscopes
These are currently under development and are mainly used to identify possible sources of blood loss.

FURTHER TESTS
Investigations for malabsorption
Xylose absorption The 5-hour urinary recovery of orally ingested xylose (non-metabolised carbohydrate) should be >25% and is abnormal if the gut mucosa is abnormal. The technique requires that normal renal function is present.

Protein absorption This is rarely assessed directly.

Fat absorption In the faecal fat test, after ingestion of 70 g of fat, normally <5 g appears in the faeces. The method requires a 3-day collection while ensuring adequate fat intake.

An alternative is the ^{14}C-linoleic acid breath test, which measures fat uptake. Radiolabelled ^{14}C-linoleic acid is given by mouth, and either the serum radioactivity measured, or exhaled $^{14}CO_2$ monitored by a breath test.

Investigation of Diarrhoea and Malabsorption

As discussed in the introductory section, it is important to define whether a patient is describing changes in consistency, frequency or volume of stool.

The causes of diarrhoea may be defined physiologically:

- Secretory (e.g. cholera toxin or hormonally-mediated neoplastic syndromes) – secretion of salt and water by gut epithelial cells.
- Exudative (e.g. inflammatory bowel disease and ulceration) – loss of interstitial fluid from the inflamed gut wall.
- Osmotic (e.g. ingestion of laxatives such as magnesium salts) – high osmotic non-absorbable substances in the gut lumen prevent water absorption. In malabsorption, non-absorbed food (e.g. fat) can contribute to osmotic load.
- Hypermotility (e.g. irritable bowel syndrome).

Often, more than one mechanism is present.

INVESTIGATION OF DIARRHOEA

Initially, it is important to elicit a clinical history in order to identify likely causes.

Small-intestinal disease

Here, there is either watery or fatty diarrhoea; often, there is no pain, though if pain occurs, it is not closely related to defaecation. The presence of blood is unusual. The stool volume may be large.

Pancreatic disease

This is classically steatorrhoea, with pale floating stools, 'oil on water' from excess fat loss. It may be associated with pancreatic pain after eating (pain in the back, or ill-defined upper abdominal pain).

Colonic cause

This is often associated with colonic pain (lower abdominal colic, below umbilicus, immediately before defaecation and is relieved by passage of stool). The stools are bloody if the condition is associated with inflammation. The stool volume is not large (only 1200 ml of fluid enters colon from terminal ileum daily).

CURRENT APPROACHES

There are two stages.

The first is to use the clinical history to localise the probable organ of involvement.

The second is to aim for an anatomical diagnosis:

- Small intestine, perhaps involving mucosal disease (e.g. coeliac) – perform duodenal biopsy.
- Pancreas, possibly cancer or pancreatitis – perform ultrasound, CT, ERCP.
- Colonic, possibly neoplasia, diverticular disease, irritable bowel syndrome, colitis – perform sigmoidoscopy/ colonoscopy/ barium enema.

Functional tests, i.e. tests of malabsorption, should be performed only if the diagnosis is obscure.

SUSPECTED SPECIFIC MALABSORPTION

Vitamin B_{12} absorption

The vitamin B_{12} absorption is complex and includes:

- Combination of ingested B_{12} with intrinsic factor in the stomach.
- Absorption of intrinsic factor B_{12} complex via specific receptors in the ileum.

In addition, the pancreas is involved in ensuring that the B_{12} intrinsic factor combination is stable. Bacteria in the small intestine may also lead to B_{12} deficiency due to bacterial utilisation of the vitamin.

Vitamin B_{12} deficiency should be suspected if:

- Previous gastric surgery has been performed, especially partial gastrectomy.
- There is ileal disease or resection.
- There is a history of autoimmune disease (leading to gastric atrophy).
- There is vitiligo (auto-immune marker) or peripheral neuropathy.

Blood tests

These include a serum assay for B_{12}. A high mean corpuscular volume (MCV), and low haemoglobin and low white cell count reflect B_{12} deficiency (or folate deficiency). Autoantibodies (anti-parietal cells, anti-intrinsic factor) indicate the presence of autoimmune disease.

Specific absorption tests

- Part I Schilling test (B_{12} alone) – abnormal in all types of B_{12} malabsorption.
- Part II Schilling test plus intrinsic factor – corrects absorption in gastric abnormality.
- Part III Schilling test (using pancreatic enzymes), corrects if there is pancreatic deficiency.
- Part IV Schilling test (after antibiotics) corrects if there is bacterial overgrowth.

Investigation of Diarrhoea and Malabsorption

Schilling tests involve ingesting radioactive B_{12}, with simultaneous injection of B_{12} to ensure that binding sites are saturated, and subsequent measurement of absorbed B_{12} by measuring % of B_{12} radioactivity appearing in urine.

LACTOSE AND OTHER CARBOHYDRATES

Upper small-intestinal enterocyte enzymes cause splitting of disaccharides (e.g. sucrose, split by sucrase, provides glucose–fructose; lactose, split by lactase, provides glucose–galactose; maltose, split by maltase, provides glucose–glucose) to monosaccharides prior to digestion. Unabsorbed disaccharides lead to diarrhoea due to unabsorbed osmotic load, while fermentation in the colon worsens diarrhoea, with excess gas production. Clinically two forms of deficiency are relevant.

- Genetic lactase deficiency: this is in fact the normal situation of loss of lactase during development after weaning. About 90% of the world's population lose lactase, in which case ingestion of sufficient milk leads to diarrhoea. Northern European populations tend to maintain the enzyme.
- Acquired lactase deficiency: occurs transiently after small-intestinal gut infections, or when other diseases (e.g. coeliac disease) lead to loss of enterocyte number and function.

Assessment

Lactose tolerance test This is a clinical test in which patients drink a solution containing 50 g of lactose. Lactase deficiency is shown by symptoms of diarrhoea developing, and by the lack of an increase in blood glucose after 30 minutes.

Breath test Here, 50 g of lactose is ingested, which in the absence of lactase and leads to an increase in breath hydrogen within 2 hours; this reflects the production by gut bacteria of hydrogen from non-absorbed lactose.

BILE ACIDS

Normally, bile acids are produced in the liver, stored in the gallbladder, and released into the duodenum via the common bile ducts after meals. After they have facilitated fat absorption by delivering triglycerides to the enterocyte surface (in the form of 'micelles'), bile acids are reabsorbed in terminal ileum, and returned to the liver. There are two degrees of bile acid malabsorption seen after ileal resection:

- Malabsorption with short ileal resection (<1 m). Some bile acids are not reabsorbed and passed into the colon, where they induce colonic secretion. Sufficient bile acid is resynthesised by the liver to maintain fat absorption normally. Treatment is by giving a bile acid-binding agent by mouth (cholestyramine).
- Larger ileal resection (>1 m). Bile acid loss is such that the liver cannot synthesise sufficient replacement, thus diminishing the bile salt pool. Inadequate bile acids are therefore present in the upper gut, so that fat absorption is incomplete and the undigested fat causes steatorrhoea. The large volume of diarrhoea and steatorrhoea is due to colonic fermentation of fat to short-chain fatty acids, which are osmotically active and induce secretion. When bile salts are deficient, there is also a change in the constitution of bile in the gallbladder, and cholesterol gallstones begin to precipitate as cholesterol is not kept in solution. Treatment of steatorrhoea due to bile salt deficiency is by fat restriction. Energy requirements can be satisfied by substituting medium-chain triglyceride oil (or normal dietary fat, although this is often poorly tolerated by patients). These MCT oils are absorbed directly into portal blood without requiring bile salts.

Abnormal bile salt metabolism can occur for reasons other than ileal disease:

- Liver disease – cholestatic liver disease (obstructive jaundice, primary biliary cirrhosis, etc.) causes decrease bile flow and fat malabsorption.
- Bacterial overgrowth in the common bile duct or upper small intestine can degrade bile acids so that they cannot facilitate fat absorption.

Diagnosis

- Support from history of ileal resection/disease or hepatobiliary disease.
- Functional testing – administration of ^{14}C-labelled glycocholic acid, which should be absorbed by the ileum and pass to the liver. If ^{14}C-glycocholic acid is exposed to bacteria (from bacterial overgrowth, or as it is lost into the colon), labelled carbon dioxide is released which can be measured in the breath. An early abnormal rise in $^{14}CO_2$ in the breath suggests the presence of bacteria in the upper gut/common bile duct. A late rise in breath $^{14}CO_2$ indicates the passage of excess bile acid to the colon in ileal disease.

Malabsorptive State

Definition
Failure to absorb properly the nutrients present in the gut.

Malabsorption should be distinguished from malnutrition, which is inadequate food intake. However, in malabsorption patients may appear malnourished.

While absorption is the main function of the small intestine, and malabsorption generally reflects small-intestinal disease, diseases in other organs may also cause malabsorption. For example, the pancreas, in failing to produce digestive enzymes, may cause chronic pancreatitis.

Malabsorption may be general for all foodstuffs (for example diffuse small-intestinal disease), or may be specific – for example, failure to absorb glucose and galactose in milk due to a lack of the enzyme lactase. Generally, the term malabsorption syndrome is limited to patients who have generalised problems with absorption. In such patients, fat malabsorption is generally the biggest problem, so the presence of steatorrhoea – excess fat in the stool – is often taken as the strongest evidence for malabsorption.

Malabsorption can arise for many reasons, which can be classified conceptually.

Conditions in the gut lumen
- Lack of pancreatic enzymes, e.g. chronic pancreatitis.
- Lack of solubilising bile salts (obstructive jaundice).
- Bacterial overgrowth.
- Inadequate mixing/intestinal hurry (motility disorders, post-gastrectomy).

Conditions in the gut wall
- Small-intestinal mucosal disease, e.g. coeliac disease, tropical sprue, Whipple's disease.
- Chronic inflammation, e.g. diffuse Crohn's disease.

Conditions outside the gut wall
- Lymphatic abnormalities, e.g. lymphoma obstructing lymphatics.

Inadequate gut length
- Short gut or short bowel syndrome after surgery.

SYMPTOMS AND SIGNS OF MALABSORPTION
Symptoms are highly variable, but diarrhoea, fatigue and weight loss are common. Signs vary from none to anaemia, pigmentation, finger clubbing (see **1**), and evidence of specific deficiencies (glossitis, cheilosis) sore corners of the mouth, hyperkeratosis, night-blindness, purpura, ecchymoses, oedema and eczema (e.g. **92**).

LONG-TERM CONSEQUENCES OF MALABSORPTION
There are a number of physiological problems in other organs following malabsorption. These include:
- Renal stones, which are of two types: (a) oxalate stones due to excess absorption of dietary oxalate if there is steatorrhoea (with steatorrhoea, there is no free calcium to produce insoluble calcium oxalate); (b) urate stones (from dehydration and a tendency to pass acid urine when diarrhoea is present).
- Osteomalacia: failure to absorb vitamin D, leading to loss of calcium from bone. This is assessed biochemically by low calcium, high phosphate, increased bony alkaline phosphatase. Radiographs indicate pseudofractures (Looser's zone, **93**), but are less sensitive.
- Night-blindness (vitamin A deficiency).
- Peripheral neuropathy (B_{12} deficiency) in ileal resection only.
- Secondary changes in the pancreas (decrease in digestive enzymes due to malnutrition).
- Gallstones (due to depleted bile salt pool leading to super saturated bile); these occur with extensive ileal resection.

Malabsorptive State

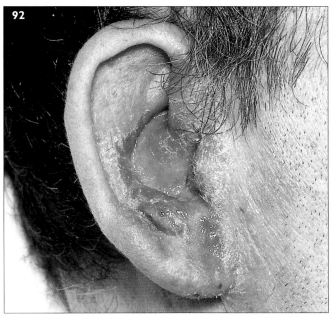

92 Chronic zinc deficiency resulting in chronic eczematous eruption.

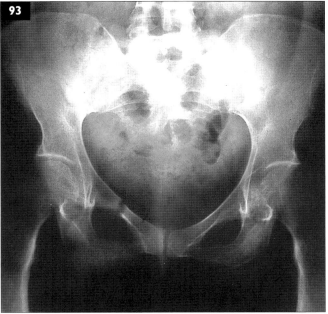

93 Osteomalacia, shown by a Looser's zone, a pseudo fracture, clearly seen in the right superior pubic ramus.

Coeliac Disease – Gluten-Sensitive Enteropathy

Definition
Inflammatory process affecting the small intestine – predominantly the duodenum and jejunum – in susceptible individuals in response to the ingestion of wheat protein (gluten and gliadin). This results in changes in small-intestinal architecture with loss of normal villous architecture and malabsorption of nutrients.

Epidemiology and aetiology
The condition occurs mainly in people of Northern European origin, though it can affect most races. It is most common in Eire, the UK and Northern Europe (1 in 1000–2500 individuals with higher prevalence figures, if populations are meticulously screened). Almost all patients carry the genetic background of possession of the HLA haplotype B8 DRQ_2; this genetic make-up probably confers the ability to mount a specific immune response to a toxic peptide in wheat protein.

Pathophysiology
In susceptible individuals, ingestion of wheat results in development of a cell and antibody-mediated immune response to peptides in wheat gliadin; this response is then expressed in the mucosa of the upper small intestine as wheat is digested. As part of the response, the turnover of epithelial cells of the intestine increases, causing loss of the normal finger-like villi and flattening of the mucosal surface – so-called villous atrophy. The surface area available for digestion falls, and the individual epithelial cells are also abnormal (**94, 95**).

Clinical history
This is very variable. In some patients the condition is manifest as soon as wheat enters the diet, i.e. on weaning, but in others it may not be apparent until late childhood or adult life. Some patients present with a full-blown malabsorption picture – diarrhoea, weight loss, anaemia and multiple vitamin deficiencies. Others may present with, for example, mild anaemia only, or secondary effects such as infertility or delayed puberty. Some patients are diagnosed on screening family members of a patient – about 10% of first-degree relatives will be affected.

Physical examination
This is also very variable. Often, there are no physical signs. In very severe cases there may be pigmentation, weight loss, short stature, delayed puberty, anaemia, glossitis, purpura, oedema, and secondary skeletal changes from long-term osteomalacia.

Laboratory and special examinations
Evidence of malabsorption There are almost invariably low folate levels, low iron and anaemia. Howell–Jolly bodies seen on the blood film reflect splenic atrophy which occurs in coeliac disease for unknown reasons. There are also abnormal coagulation tests, low serum albumen and low serum calcium in severe cases. Serum alkaline phosphatase activity is high if bone disease is present. The conventional diagnostic test is histopathology of upper small intestine – duodenal biopsy taken at endoscopy or (less frequently nowadays) jejunal biopsy (small-intestinal biopsy – 'Crosby capsule').

Blood tests 'Anti-endomysial antibodies' are almost specific and may in due time replace biopsy tests in clinical practice. The antibody is a component of smooth muscle cells. 'Anti-gliadin' and 'anti-gluten' are non-specific unless in sophisticated form to detect IgA class antibodies.

Radiology Small-intestinal radiographs (small bowel enema or barium flow-through) may show abnormal mucosal pattern and thickening of jejunal folds (**96**), though they are not specific for coeliac disease. In mild disease appearances may be normal. In severe, long-standing disease the changes may be prominent and extend also into the ileum.

Special forms
Childhood and adult coeliac disease differ. In childhood, there is a possibility that gluten sensitivity may be transient, and after a time gluten may be reintroduced safely. This, however, is rare even in childhood, and does not seem to occur in the adult.

Occasionally, adult patients do not respond despite proper dietary therapy (see below). This is loosely called non-responsive coeliac disease.

Coeliac Disease – Gluten-Sensitive Enteropathy

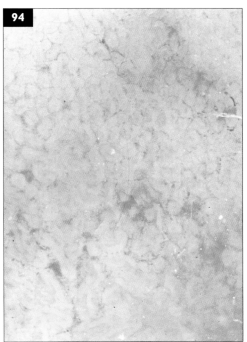

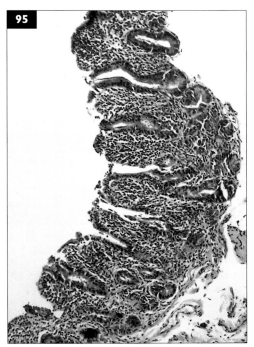

94 Flat jejunal biopsy under dissecting microscope showing no villi and only crypts in coeliac disease.

95 Histopathology of coeliac disease, showing flat mucosa, and chronic inflammation.

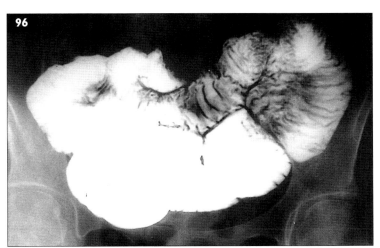

96 Coeliac disease on barium follow through – note the valvulae conniventes are thickened and straight in the jejunum.

Coeliac Disease – Gluten-Sensitive Enteropathy

Dermatitis herpetiformis This is a skin condition presenting with a highly itchy eruption on skin – typically the elbows. Most patients, even if gut symptoms are absent, have a gluten-sensitive enteropathy. Skin and gut improve with withdrawal of gluten from the diet. The condition involves deposition of IgA in the skin.

Differential diagnosis
Differentiate from other causes of malabsorption and small-intestinal inflammation:
- In childhood, other food-sensitive enteropathies, i.e. milk-sensitivity.
- In adults, Crohn's disease of small intestine, lymphoma, Whipple's disease.

Prognosis
Treated childhood coeliac disease has an excellent prognosis, provided that dietary treatment is adequate. The gut mucosa returns to normal.

In adults, response may be only partial, with minor continuing histological abnormality although malabsorption resolves. Long-term complications in adult disease include:

- Small-intestinal lymphoma.
- Development of ulceration of intestine.
- Small-intestinal cancer.
- Cancers elsewhere (e.g. oesophagus) are also more common.

These complications are discussed below.

Management
Dietary treatment involves the institution of a gluten-free diet. Patient education and dietician support is vital. Many prepared foods contain unsuspected gluten. A gluten-free diet avoids wheat, wheat products and rye. Oats and barley are questionable. Rice is permitted.

When disease is very severe, resolution of the intestinal inflammation can be helped by corticosteroids. If response is poor despite strict gluten withdrawal, oral azathioprine may help.

Follow-up This is important. Checking for early return of deficiencies (Hb, folate, Fe levels) may give early warning of inadequate dietary compliance or complication.

Complications of Coeliac Disease

Complications include those found at presentation and those that may occur at any time.

Those at presentation are generally the consequences of malabsorption, e.g. anaemia, and not specific to coeliac disease.

Other complications include:
- Failure to improve after gluten withdrawal, or relapse after treatment. This is most often due to failure to adhere to the diet – knowingly or unknowingly.
- Development of ulcerative ileojejunitis (**97, 98**).
- Development of lymphoma.
- Development of small-intestinal cancer.

Non-specific ileojejunitis
This is a rare condition, in which ulceration of the jejunum and ileum occurs (non-granulomatous, distinguishing it from Crohn's disease). Symptoms include pain, malabsorption, bleeding, obstruction and perforation. In some patients there may be an underlying lymphoma of the small intestine, but this is not always present.

Treatment is difficult – both strict gluten withdrawal and corticosteroids are used.

Small-intestinal lymphoma
In adults (but not children), 1–3% of individuals will develop a lymphoma due to a malignant T-cell clone arising in the small-intestinal mucosa. Patients present with diarrhoea, weight loss, anaemia, bleeding or perforation/obstruction. Laparotomy may be needed to achieve diagnosis. Chemotherapy is generally ineffective and the prognosis is poor. The chances of developing lymphoma fall if patients adhere to a gluten-free diet.

Carcinoma
There is an increased incidence of carcinoma in a number of sites in patients with coeliac disease, a complication again restricted to adults. The risk reduces after gluten withdrawal. Jejunal tumours (presenting with anaemia, obstruction or frank bleeding) and oesophageal tumours (presenting with dysphagia) are the most common sites.

Complications of Coeliac Disease

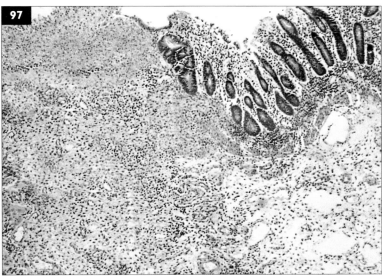

97 Histological section in ulcerative ileojejunitis, showing loss of mucosal epithelium and ulcer formation.

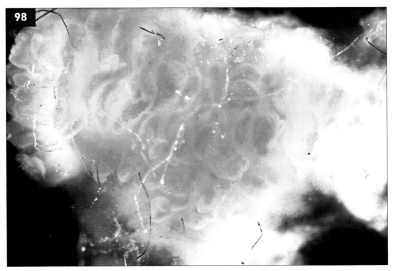

98 Dissecting microscopic appearance in ulcerative ileojejunitis.

Whipple's Disease – Intestinal Lipodystrophy

Definition
An infection with the organism *Trophyrema whipellii*, which can affect most organs of the body, generally diagnosed when malabsorption occurs, with a characteristic macrophage-rich inflammation of the small-intestinal mucosa (**99, 100**).

Epidemiology and aetiology
A rare condition, characteristically but not exclusively affecting middle-aged Caucasian males. The recently described Actinomycete, *Trophyrema whippelii* (**101**), can be identified in affected tissues. The mode of transmission and basis of susceptibility is unknown.

Pathophysiology
Affected tissues contain bacteria, and become infiltrated with macrophages. In the intestine, the lymphatics can become blocked, and the normal villous architecture is destroyed, causing malabsorption. Other effects include joint swelling, pleural and pericardial inflammation, central nervous system and meningeal involvement.

Clinical history
Most patients have a history of intermittent arthritis. The diagnosis is usually made when diarrhoea and malabsorption develop. Pleurisy, cardiac involvement (conduction defects, valve problems), and fits and ophthalmoplegia are rare complications.

Physical examination
At diagnosis, pigmentation, clubbing, and other evidence of advanced malabsorption are usually present. Lymphadenopathy, synovial thickening, heart signs, and cranial nerve abnormalities may be present.

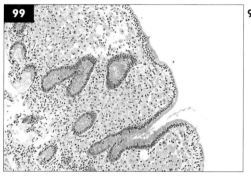

99 Histological section of small intestine in Whipple's disease, with foamy macrophages filling the mucosal space and the lack of normal villous architecture.

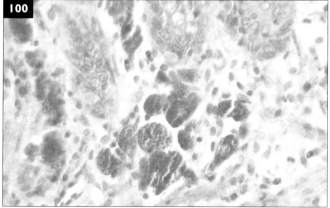

100 Periodic acid–Schiff (PAS)-positive (magenta colour) material characteristic of Whipple's disease in the small intestinal biopsy.

Whipple's Disease – Intestinal Lipodystrophy

Laboratory and special examinations

Diagnosis is most commonly made by examination of small-intestinal histology. A molecular biological approach using the polymerase chain reaction (PCR) is needed to identify the bacterium, amplifying bacterial RNA, as the organism is very difficult to culture. This is not necessary for clinical management. Small-intestinal radiograph shows a characteristic dilated appearance (102). Anaemia, folate deficiency, and blood tests indicative of malabsorption will be found.

Differential diagnosis

Differentiate from other causes of malabsorption.

Prognosis

Good if treated early with appropriate antibiotics. Relapsing forms may occur – perhaps indicating the development of antibiotic resistance. Central nervous system and cardiac valve abnormalities do not necessarily reverse after treatment.

Management options

Early and prolonged antibiotic therapy is required. Antibiotics should initially be able to pass the blood–brain barrier, e.g. penicillin and streptomycin, or co-trimoxazole, followed by up to a year's oral therapy, e.g. co-trimoxazole, tetracycline.

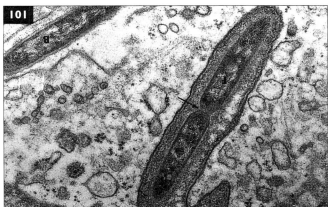

101 Electron microscopic picture showing the Whipple's bacillus – *Trophyrema whippelii.*

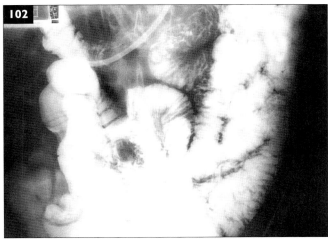

102 Small bowel enema in a patient with Whipple's disease, showing dilated bowel with thickening of the valvulae conniventes.

Short Gut or Short Bowel Syndrome

Definition
Clinical problems arising from reduced intestinal length, following massive intestinal resection (**103**).

Epidemiology and aetiology
In children, the syndrome results generally from surgery for congenital disorders (volvulus, adhesions). In adults, it follows trauma, thrombosis of vessels, or Crohn's disease (generally following multiple operations).

Pathophysiology
The pathophysiology is complex. Two major types may be distinguished:
• Loss of small intestine only.
• Loss of small intestine plus substantial loss of colon.

In the latter group, intestinal problems due to loss of absorptive capacity are worsened by dehydration due to loss of water-reabsorbing function of colon.

Small gut syndrome (SGS) generally does not occur if more than half of the length of the small intestine remains (initial length approximately 5 metres in adults). If <1 m remains, SGS is severe and enteral feeding inadequate. Loss of jejunum is less serious than loss of ileum (the ileum can adapt to take on jejunal functions, but jejunum cannot take over specific ileal functions such as B_{12} and bile salt absorption).

Malabsorption in SGS is due to:
• Loss of absorbing capacity.
• Presence of undigested fat in intestinal lumen impairing absorption of other nutrients (e.g. calcium, magnesium).
• Bacterial overgrowth.

Clinical history
The surgical history is obvious, but surgical details are important. Patients with surgically created 'blind loops' in addition to resection are more prone to bacterial overgrowth. Knowledge of the extent of resection and associated colonic loss will define which patients will eventually be able to live without parenteral supplementation, or whether this is impossible.

Physical examination
Signs of malabsorption, dehydration, and precipitating disease may be present.

Laboratory and special examinations
In SGS, vitamin and mineral deficiencies may develop slowly over years, so magnesium, zinc, copper, selenium, and vitamins A, D, E and K should be considered. It is useful to document the amount of fat in the stools. Barium follow-through allows measurement of residual intestine, and definition of the presence of strictures and blind loops.

Differential diagnosis
None – although in conditions like Crohn's disease, both disease in the residual small intestine and the lack of length contribute to the severity of the syndrome.

Prognosis
The prognosis is variable. If >1.5 m of small intestine remains there is a problem in maintaining bodyweight, but it should be possible to maintain near-normal nutrition on a normal diet. If <1 m of small intestine remains, there will be severe problems with malabsorption and weight loss; dehydration will also be a problem if there is ileostomy or substantial colonic loss. In this group, total parenteral nutrition is often necessary, and this produces its own risk of sepsis and catheter problems.

Management
In the initial stage, parenteral fluid and electrolyte replacement is necessary and, if severe, total parenteral nutrition to prevent excessive weight loss. Some oral feeding may be necessary to prevent gut atrophy.

In the subsequent stage, it must be assessed whether adequate fluid and food intake can be maintained orally. Frequent solid food, low lactose and low fat, and calorie supplementation with medium-chain triglycerides, and anti-motility agents is required. If this is inadequate, total parenteral nutrition will be required.

Complications
Complications are generally related to malabsorption. Renal stones (oxalate) (**104**) occur if the colon is intact due to increased absorption of dietary oxalate. Gallstones occur due to bile salt depletion. Specific vitamin deficiencies include: osteomalacia (vitamin D), night-blindness (vitamin A) and peripheral neuropathy (vitamin E).

Short Gut or Short Bowel Syndrome

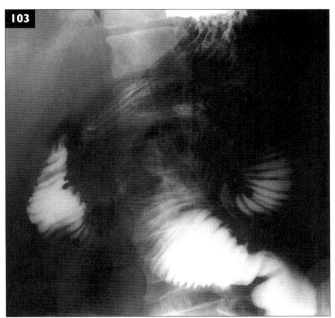

103 Short gut. This barium study shows the stomach, duodenum, 25 cm of jejunum and distal colon in continuity, after surgery for ischaemia.

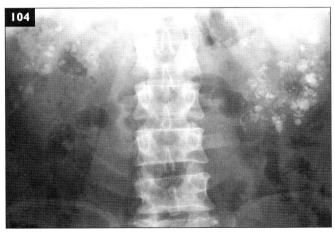

104 Bilateral punctate calcification on both kidneys.

Protein-Losing Enteropathy

Definition
A variety of gastrointestinal conditions cause protein loss into the gut, leading to weight loss, and hypoalbuminaemia. Loss may occur through ulcerated areas, as in inflammatory conditions, or through loss of intestinal lymph as in lymphangiectasia (**105**). A protein-losing enteropathy (PLE) may be only one aspect of an inflammatory or neoplastic condition affecting the gut, or as in intestinal lymphangiectasia may be the predominant problem. The causes of PLE are as follows:
* Disorders of the lymphatics – primary lymphangiectasia (familial or sporadic). Secondary intestinal lymphangiectasia (blockage of lymphatic flow by tumour, infection, e.g. tuberculosis, retroperitoneal fibrosis or inflammation).
* Inflammation and ulcerative conditions. In the stomach, Ménétrier's disease, Zollinger–Ellison syndrome; in the small intestine, coeliac disease, tropical sprue, allergic gastroenteropathy, vasculitis and Crohn's disease.

Pathophysiology
This varies with the site of protein loss. When loss is from the stomach, symptoms only occur when the liver cannot increase albumin synthesis sufficient to maintain plasma oncotic pressure, so oedema occurs. In these circumstances, absorption from the small intestine is normal so nutrition is generally maintained. In small-intestinal lymphangiectasia, loss of fluid from dilated lymphatic channels (lacteals) leads to hypoalbuminaemia, hypogammaglobulinaemia, and leakage of long-chain fatty acids because dilated lymphatics rupture into intestine (**106, 107**). Lymphocyte loss (T-cells) also occurs. Patients develop steatorrhoea and diarrhoea, and are susceptible to infections.

Clinical history
Symptoms are:
* Characteristic of primary cause (e.g. pain and diarrhoea with Crohn's disease, anorexia and weight loss with gastric cancer).
* Low plasma proteins cause oedema.
* Malabsorption (if part of intestinal lymphangiectasia).

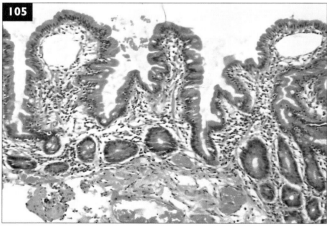

105 Intestinal biopsy showing lymphangiectasia – dilated lymphatic spaces at the tips of the villi.

Protein-Losing Enteropathy

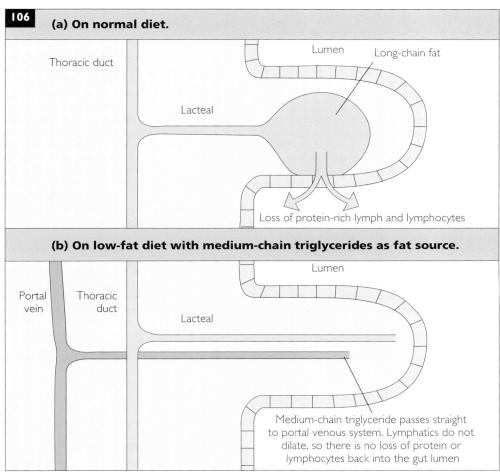

(a) On normal diet.

Thoracic duct

Lumen   Long-chain fat

Lacteal

Loss of protein-rich lymph and lymphocytes

(b) On low-fat diet with medium-chain triglycerides as fat source.

Lumen

Portal vein   Thoracic duct

Lacteal

Medium-chain triglyceride passes straight to portal venous system. Lymphatics do not dilate, so there is no loss of protein or lymphocytes back into the gut lumen

106 Mechanism of protein loss in lymphangiectasia.

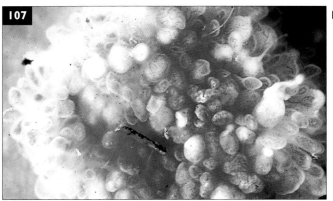

107 Dissecting microscopic appearances of lymphangiectatic intestinal mucosa. Note the fat-dilated and leaking lymphatics.

Protein-Losing Enteropathy

Physical signs

Oedema, and other evidence of malabsorption. In intestinal lymphangiectasia, there may be other lymphatic abnormalities, such as long-standing peripheral lymphoedema (**108**).

Laboratory examinations

Hypoalbuminaemia and hypogamma-globu-linaemia occur, in the absence of liver disease or renal loss. In intestinal lymphangiectasia there is a low circulating lymphocyte count. To prove the extent of PLE, dynamic tests are required to document the loss of an intravenously injected isotope (i.e. ^{51}Cr-labelled albumin) and based on faecal collection. Anatomical studies are required to identify the nature and site of protein loss. Endoscopy and barium meal will demonstrate lesions in the stomach (thickened folds of Ménétrier's disease, gastric lymphoma or hypersecretory syndromes). Small-intestine radiograph studies may show:

- Generalised oedema reflecting hypo-proteinaemia.
- Characteristic signs of lymphoedema.

Jejunal biopsies show characteristic lymphatic dilatation.

Differential diagnosis

PLE is generally part of another syndrome. In intestinal lymphoma, differential diagnosis is between the primary and secondary causes. CT scanning will exclude mesenteric or retroperitoneal lymphadenopathy. Peripheral lymphoangiography will identify peripheral lymphatic abnormalities.

Prognosis

If part of an associated condition, then prognosis of that condition should be considered. Primary lymphangiectasia presenting in childhood may be very severe, and even with dietary management, patients may remain with malabsorption and be prone to infection.

Management

If part of an associated condition, then management of that condition should be considered. In Ménétrier's disease, anti-inflammatory drugs have been tried with little effect and in severe cases gastrectomy has been used. In small-intestinal lymphangiectasia, disease is occasionally limited to small segments, so surgery can be performed, but this is infrequent. If not, dietary treatment is the main approach, in particular a strict low-fat diet, with medium-chain triglycerides to provide calories (this form of fat does not pass through lacteals, see **106**) and identification and treatment of deficiencies.

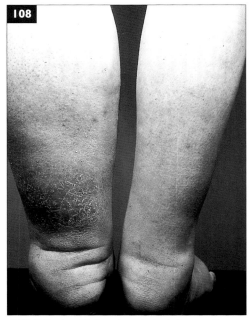

108 Patients with lymphangiectasia frequently have peripheral lymphatic abnormalities leading to asymmetric oedema of the legs.

Tropical Sprue; Post-Infectious Malabsorption

Definition
This is acute or chronic diarrhoea and malabsorption, occurring in the developing world, and associated with abnormal small-intestinal mucosal structure. It is probably attributable to infection. Two forms are distinguished – acute and chronic.

Epidemiology and aetiology
Acute epidemics of sprue affecting whole villages are reported in Asia, probably following acute infections. Chronic tropical sprue was most often recognised in expatriates living in developing countries. Viral infections may initiate acute sprue, and in chronic sprue bacterial infection may be responsible. The distinction between the two forms is not absolute, and traveller's malabsorption seen for example in overland hikers returning from Asia may be part of the same spectrum.

Pathophysiology
There are abnormalities in the small-intestinal mucosa leading to malabsorption. Severe folate deficiency may prevent the mucosa from undergoing its normal proliferative cycle.

Clinical history
Acute sprue describes the emergence of prolonged diarrhoea, with varying degrees of malabsorption, after an acute diarrhoeal illness. Chronic sprue may present insidiously with diarrhoea, weight loss and anaemia, sometimes after returning to a temperate climate.

Physical examination
Signs of malabsorption and weight loss may be present.

Laboratory and special examinations
Attempts must be made by routine techniques to culture single pathogens. There may be laboratory evidence of malabsorption and resulting deficiencies. Anaemia with macrocytosis and folate deficiency are generally present.

The most specific test is small-intestinal biopsy which shows abnormal villous architecture, with varying degrees of flattening of the villous pattern (rarely as severe as in coeliac disease). It is important to realise that any dweller in the tropics may have deviations from the normal western-type villous pattern of finger-like mucosal projections, and minor abnormalities and predominantly leaf-like villi may be the norm (109).

Differential diagnosis
Differentiate from other malabsorptive states such as coeliac disease, and from single-agent infections such as giardiasis. Persistent diarrhoea with no evidence of malabsorption after acute gastroenteritis may merely be post-infectious irritable bowel.

Management options and prognosis
Antibiotic therapy (e.g. tetracycline for 2 weeks) plus folic acid replacement (for some months) is recommended. In severe cases, replacement of other deficiencies may be required. Parasitic infestation such as giardiasis may require specific antimicrobial treatment (e.g. metronidazole).

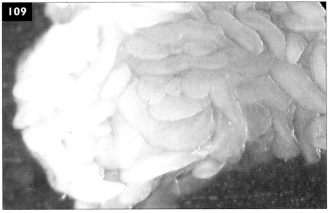

109 Dissecting microscopic appearance showing leaf-like villi.

Bacterial Overgrowth

Definition
Bacterial colonisation of the small intestine leading to malabsorption of one or more nutrients.

Aetiology and epidemiology
Uncommon condition which occurs in the presence of: (a) anatomical abnormality in the small intestine; or (b) rarely, functional abnormality of immune defence.
The anatomical predisposing causes are:
- Jejunal diverticulosis (**110**).
- Previous surgery causing blind loops.
- Crohn's disease when subacute obstruction or enteroenteric fistulae are present.
- Pseudo-obstruction due to motility disorders.
- Infiltration or degenerative disorders affecting motility (e.g. systemic sclerosis (**111**), amyloidosis.
Functional causes include:
- Loss of gastric acidity (pernicious anaemia, long-term acid-suppressive therapy), which removes generalised first-line of defence against ingested bacteria.
- Immunodeficiency syndrome (e.g. hypo-gammaglobulinaemia, HIV).

Pathophysiology
The upper small intestine is normally sterile except for transient passage of ingested bacteria. Colonisation occurs when 10^6/ml or more bacteria are found on duodenal or small-intestinal aspiration. Bacteria cause diarrhoea in a number of ways:
- Bile salt deconjugation leads to fat malabsorption.
- Nutrient uptake by bacteria leads to deficiencies (e.g. vitamin B_{12} deficiency), and rarely hypoproteinaemia following loss of essential amino acids.
  Rarely, as in the patient with a jejuno-ileal bypass for morbid obesity, in whom a large blind loop (the majority of the small intestine) is present, an immune response to the bacteria can induce systemic symptoms of arthritis and skin lesions (**112**).

Clinical history
Episodes of diarrhoea, or chronic diarrhoea; history of a response to antibiotics is often helpful.

Laboratory and specialised examinations
To establish a diagnosis of bacterial overgrowth it is desirable to demonstrate:

- The cause (generally anatomical).
- The presence of bacteria.
- A response to antibiotics.
Difficulties in satisfying these criteria may arise because the techniques for demonstrating the presence of bacteria are not satisfactory, because culture of bacteria is difficult to achieve, and recolonisation takes place rapidly after treatment.
  To demonstrate the cause – use a barium follow-through (see **111**).
  To demonstrate the presence of bacteria, use:
- Functional tests (breath hydrogen test, ^{14}C-glycocholic acid breath test) (**113**).
- Urinary indicans (bacterial metabolites).
- Direct intubation, counting and culture (this needs full bacteriological facilities, particularly for culture of anaerobes).

Special tests Occasionally, sophisticated tests of gastrointestinal immune system (measuring IgA levels in blood and IgA cells in mucosa) may be needed.

Differential diagnosis
Differentiate from other malabsorption syndromes.

Prognosis
Generally not a severe condition unless it has been unrecognised for a long time and complications such as peripheral neuropathy, due to B_{12} deficiency have occurred.

Management
Occasionally, blind loops may require surgical correction, but more often intermittent courses of antibiotics are helpful. Repeated episodes of antibiotic treatment, however, may be needed. Empirical regimes include short courses of:
- Tetracyclines.
- Metronidazole.
- Ciprofloxacin.
- Erythromycin.

Bacterial Overgrowth

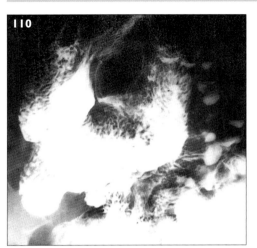

110 Multiple jejunal diverticula containing fluid levels, in a patient with bacterial overgrowth and who had peripheral neuropathy as a consequence.

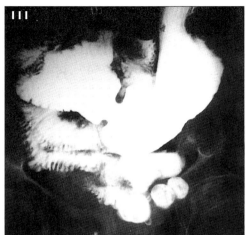

111 Barium meal and follow-through in a patient with systemic sclerosis, showing dilated hypomotile intestine, a breeding ground for bacterial overgrowth.

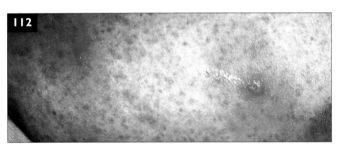

112 Part of the 'arthritis dermatitis' syndrome seen in a patient with jejunoileal bypass This is probably an immune reaction to bacterial overgrowth.

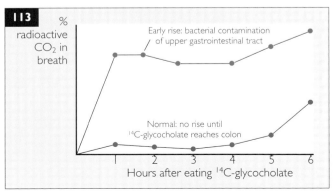

113 ^{14}C-glycocholate breath test to detect bacterial overgrowth.

Radiation Enteritis

Definition
Inflammation of the intestine as a result of therapeutic irradiation. Acute radiation enteritis occurs at the time of radiation, but chronic damage may occur from months to many years afterwards.

Aetiology, epidemiology and diagnosis
This is generally seen in middle-aged and elderly females (after radiation of carcinoma of the cervix and uterus), or in elderly males (carcinoma of the prostate). It is more likely to occur with:
• High doses of radiation.
• Radiation after previous surgery (adhesions lead to fixed bowel in radiation field).
• Genetic susceptibility.
Irradiation leads to chromosomal breakage, cell death and secondary fibrosis and vasculitis.

Pathophysiology
In acute radiation enteritis, loss of mucosal cells and enhanced motility contribute to diarrhoea. In chronic cases, fibrosis (114) and local ischaemia secondary to vasculitis lead to mucosal damage, stricturing and/or fistula formation.

Clinical history
In acute radiation enteritis, nausea and diarrhoea occur during, and for some weeks after, irradiation. Diarrhoea may be fairly severe, but is generally mild and well tolerated. Chronic radiation enteritis affecting the colon, presents with diarrhoea, pain and bleeding. Symptoms are diarrhoea, pain and malabsorption when the small intestine is involved. Symptoms may be delayed for up to 20 years post-irradiation. In association, radiation cystitis may occur with frequent urinary tract infections.

Physical examination
Generally, there are cutaneous signs of irradiation (pigmentation and telangiectasia) in the abdominal field. Weight loss and signs of malabsorption may be seen.

Laboratory and specialised examinations
Acute radiation enteritis is generally self-limited and needs no investigation. The predominant aim of investigation in chronic enteritis is to define the severity and extent of radiation damage. For small-intestinal disease, radiographic examination (intubated enema or follow-through) can be used to define narrowing and structuring and irregularity in mucosa. CT scans and magnetic resonance imaging also help investigate fistulae. Serum B_{12} levels are generally low after pelvic irradiation due to damage to the terminal ileum. For suspected colonic damage, use barium enema and colonoscopy; the prime site is the rectosigmoid, so limited investigation is often all that is needed. Irradiated tissue may be friable; biopsy is diagnostic when histology shows fibroblast and vasculitis.

Differential diagnosis
The most important is local recurrence of original cancer.
 See also Radiation Colitis (p. 160).

Management
Acute radiation is managed expectantly; management of chronic radiation may be very difficult. There is no specific medical treatment for small-intestinal radiation enteritis, other than management of diarrhoea and malabsorption with anti-motility agents, replacement of deficiencies and, if severe steatorrhoea is present, the introduction of a low-fat diet. Mild colitis may improve with local corticosteroids and 5-ASA as for ulcerative colitis, but these are often not effective. With narrowing of the gut lumen by fibrous stricture, a low-residue diet may help. Surgery requires great care. Resectional surgery can be performed for local disease – the main consideration is to ensure that two ends of the bowel with residual irradiation damage are not reanastomosed.

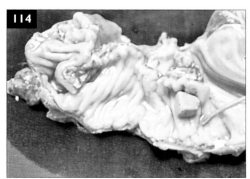

114 Resection specimen of radiation fibrosis. An enterolith (stony collection) has formed above a stricture.

Immunodeficiency States

Definition
Clinical syndromes reflecting loss of gastro-intestinal immune function. The gastrointestinal disease generally results from inability to control infection.

Aetiology and epidemiology
This is very varied. The condition may be genetic or acquired, and affect different arms of the immune system. Loss of antibodies occurs in X-linked agammaglobulinaemia, common variable immunodeficiency, IgA deficiency. Loss of T-cell function occurs in ataxia telangiectsia. Loss of both T-cell and antibody function leads to severe combined immunodeficiency. HIV disease leads to a wide variety of gastrointestinal infections (*Table 2*).

Pathophysiology
Normally, there is a highly specialised gut immune system consisting of:
- A surface layer of secretory IgA of the gut mucosa, specialised to resist digestion, providing protective immunity against gut flora.
- Cell-mediated immunity consisting of T-cells, between epithelial cells and in the lamina propria.
- Plasma cells, mainly IgA, producing IgA which can be transported to the surface of the mucosa as secretory IgA.

Table 2. Main HIV-associated infections within the gastrointestinal tract	
Mouth	• Candida • Hairy oral leukoplakia (EBV-related) • Herpes simplex (HSV) types I and II • Idiopathic ulceration
Oesophagus	• Candida oesophagitis • EBV-related ulceration • Cytomegalovirus (CMV) ulcers • HSV
Small bowel	• HIV enteropathy • *Mycobacterium avium intracellulare* complex • Giardiasis • Cryptosporidium • Microsporidium • Isospora
Liver	• *Mycobacterium avium intracellulare* complex and tuberculosis • Hepatitis B • Hepatitis C
Biliary tract	• Sclerosing cholangitis • CMV • Cryptosporidiosis • Microsporidiosis
Colon	• Colitis • CMV • Campylobacter • *Clostridium difficile* • Salmonella • *Mycobacterium avium intracellulare* complex and tuberculosis • Blastocystis hominis
Proctitis/perianal	• HSV • CMV • Warts
General	In addition, tumours (Kaposi's sarcoma, lymphoma) may occur in any site

Immunodeficiency States

Deficiencies may occur as a result of a genetic inability to produce IgA deficiency, acquired ability to make all classes of immunoglobulin (common variable hypogammaglobulinaemia), inability to make new immune responses (loss of helper T-cells in AIDS), or destruction of immunocompetent cells (chemotherapy). Often, gastrointestinal manifestations of immunodeficiency coexist with generalised immunodeficiency (e.g. recurrent chest and sinus infections).

Clinical history
For immunoglobulin deficiency, check for a history of other systemic infections. Look also for risk factors for AIDS, and/or a history of AIDS-related infections (e.g. oesophageal candidiasis).

Physical examination
In childhood, recurrent infections lead to poor development, weight loss and malabsorption. Systemic immunodeficiencies may give rise to skin infections; Kaposi's sarcoma in AIDS.

Special investigations
Check stool cultures and cultures of jejunal juice for infections. HIV antibody testing.

Check serum immunoglobulins, lymphocyte count, T-cell count, jejunal biopsy and staining for IgA, IgG and IgM. Perform a small-bowel enema – in common variable hypogamma-globulinaemia there may be nodular lymphoid hyperplasia reflecting abnormal aggregates of lymphatic cells (**115, 116**). Direct inspection of biopsies for infections (e.g. giardiasis (**117**), cryptosporidiosis (**118**).

Prognosis
This is variable. In HIV infection, eradicating gut infection is difficult. In IgA deficiency, symptoms may be mild and transient. In severe cases of combined variable immunodeficiency – T-cell deficiencies in children, retarded growth and malnutrition may occur, reflecting malabsorption.

Management
Priorities include:
- Investigation of the underlying cause.
- Culture and biopsy to identify treatable organisms.

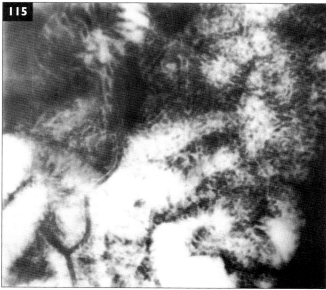

115 Small-intestinal follow-through, showing multiple nodular filling defects in the small intestine – nodular lymphoid hyperplasia, in common variable hypogammaglobulinaemia.

Immunodeficiency States

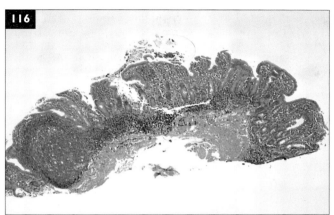

116 Small-intestinal biopsy in common variable hypogammaglobulinaemia and nodular lymphoid hyperplasia, showing prominent lymphoid follicle.

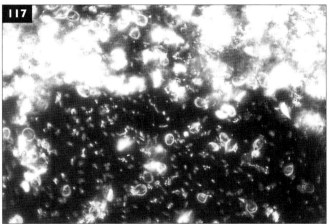

117 Dark-field view of upper intestinal contents in a patient with common variable hypergammaglobulinaemia – small 'tennis racket' outlines of *Giardia lamblia*.

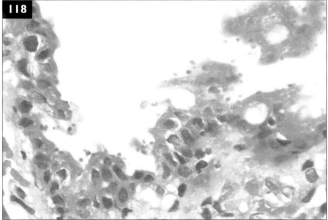

118 *Cryptosporidia* – round protozoa at the epithelial surface.

Crohn's Disease

Definition
Chronic and relapsing inflammatory disease affecting any part of intestine – generally the distal ileum and colon – of unknown aetiology. Inflammation can extend through all areas of the gut wall, and about 60% of cases include granulomatous inflammation (**119**).

Aetiology and epidemiology
More common in Northern Europe and North America than in Southern Europe or developing countries. Commences at any age, but peak in the teens to age 30, followed by a late peak in the elderly. The aetiology is unknown. Most evidence favours abnormal immune responses – overexpression of inflammatory responses against antigens (bacteria, viruses, food or autoantigens) in the gastrointestinal tract. Other theories include specific infectious agents (candidates include atypical mycobacterium, measles), but there is no agreement. There are families with several affected relatives. There is an excess of smokers among patients with Crohn's disease.

Pathophysiology
Inflammation of the gut in Crohn's leads to oedema, mucosal thickening, surface ulceration, and often fibrosis of gut wall (**120**). In the small intestine, these processes can lead to diarrhoea (due to malabsorption, particularly if bile acid malabsorption occurs in the terminal ileum), pain (from inflamed bowel irritating the peritoneum and from obstruction to passage of luminal contents due to oedema and fibrosis), and weight loss. In the colon, inflammation causes exudative bloody diarrhoea. Systemic reactions to the inflammation lead to extra-intestinal manifestations affecting joints, skin and eye.

Clinical history
Symptoms may be present for many years – typically three to four – before diagnosis is made. Non-specific symptoms include malaise, weight loss, extra-intestinal symptoms (at some time in 25–35% of cases) including arthritis (small and medium-sized joints), spondylitis, iritis, conjunctivitis, skin lesions (erythema nodosum and pyoderma gangrenosum), and aphthous ulceration of the mouth. In 15–20% of cases there will be a family history.

Small-intestinal disease usually presents with colicky pain, diarrhoea, abdominal tenderness (particularly in the right iliac fossa as the terminal ileum area is most often involved) and weight loss.

Colonic disease presents with diarrhoea, either bloody or watery, but often similar to that in ulcerative colitis.

Up to one-third of patients will have peri-anal problems (fistulae, abscesses) at some time.

With time, Crohn's disease of the terminal ileum leads to narrowing of the small intestine, and repeated episodes of subacute obstruction (**121**). This symptom can reflect either a fibrous stricture or active inflammation – deciding which is a common clinical problem. If surgery is performed (see below), removing the affected area of terminal ileum, there is a 50% chance that symptomatic inflammation will return over 5 years (often less) and that repeat surgery will be needed in about 10 years.

Investigations
A full spectrum of radiological, histological, endoscopic and general studies should be made. Crohn's disease can affect any part of the gastro-intestinal tract, although the most common pattern is: terminal ileal disease (one-third of patients), ileocaecal disease (40–50%), and colonic (20%).

General studies Full blood count, profile. To identify inflammation – ESR, C-reactive protein, low serum albumin. To identify deficiencies – B_{12} (notably in terminal ileal disease), folate, iron. If weight loss exists, malabsorption screening may be indicated. Severe malabsorption suggests diffuse jejunal disease (5% of patients).

Physical examination
Often, there are no abnormalities on examination. Possible findings include: anaemia, spondylitis, pigmentation, clubbing, perianal abscesses and fistulae, abdominal masses and cutaneous fistulae.

Special investigations
For terminal ileal disease or ileocaecal disease – small bowel enema or barium follow-through (**121, 122**), colonoscopy ± terminal ileum and caecal biopsy (**123**).

Crohn's Disease

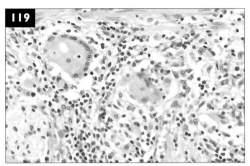

119 Two large giant cells in the submucosa in a patient with Crohn's disease.

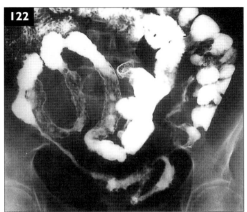

122 Classical diffuse terminal ileal Crohn's disease, with a long narrowed segment (string sign) extending over at least 60 cm Note also small 'rose-thorn' ulcers best seen in the pelvis.

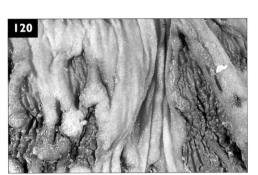

120 Macroscopic appearances of resected small intestine in Crohn's disease showing linear ulceration with unaffected areas in between.

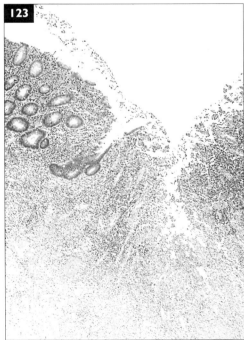

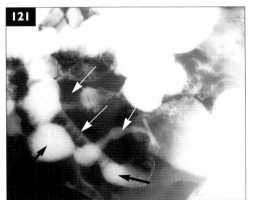

121 Extensive distal small intestinal Crohn's disease with multiple areas of narrowing (white arrows) and dilatation (black arrows) in the terminal ileum, seen on barium follow-through.

123 Histological section of small intestine showing deep fissuring ulceration and inflammation in Crohn's disease.

Crohn's Disease

For suspected colonic disease – barium enema (**124, 125**), colonoscopy(**126, 127**) and biopsy.

For suspected gastroduodenal disease – upper gastrointestinal endoscopy (**128**).

Alternative techniques include:

• White cell scanning – identifies areas of inflammation.

• Ultrasound – can identify thickening of bowel wall.

• CT or magnetic resonance imaging – identifies bowel-thickening abscesses, fistulae.

SPECIAL TYPES OF CROHN'S DISEASE
Fistulae
These can occur between any parts of the gut, i.e. ileoileal, ileocolonic, gastrocolic; between gut and other organs, i.e. bladder (**129**); or between the skin and gut – enterocutaneous.

Ileoileal fistulae may be asymptomatic, but predispose to bacterial overgrowth. Ileovesical fistulae cause urinary infection and pneumaturia. Cologastric fistulae cause vomiting, severe diarrhoea, and weight loss.

Abscesses
These may develop from local the gut through fissures in the diseased gut wall. Like fistulae, they most commonly occur above areas of stenosis. Free perforation rarely occurs. They may be a cause of high fever and discomfort, and the differential diagnosis is usually from active inflammation in the bowel wall; the two can also coexist.

Diffuse jejunal Crohn's disease
This can present with weight loss, iron deficiency, hypocalcaemia and protein-losing enteropathy.

Gastric Crohn's disease
This is generally found coincidentally on biopsy (15% of cases).

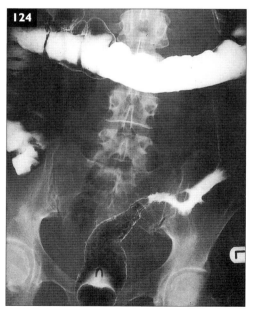

124 Barium enema in Crohn's disease showing narrowing, inflammation and deep fissuring 'rose-thorn' ulcers in the descending colon, and asymmetrical involvement (loss of haustral pattern) in the transverse colon.

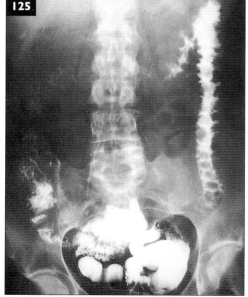

125 Extensive involvement of the descending colon with deep 'rose-thorn' ulcers in Crohn's disease.

Crohn's Disease

Duodenal Crohn's disease
This may mimic peptic ulceration, and be prone to stenose or, very rarely, bleed.

Perianal fistulae
These occur very frequently. Low perianal fistulae (internal opening below the internal anal sphincter) are relatively straightforward – local infection, discharge and pain. High perianal fistulae, particularly if overtreated surgically, may destroy the anal sphincter mechanism. Perianal fistulae may respond to antibiotics – particularly metronidazole or ciprofloxacin – but if severe or recurrent, or

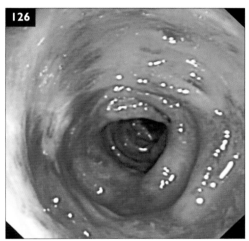

126 Patchy inflammation in the colon.

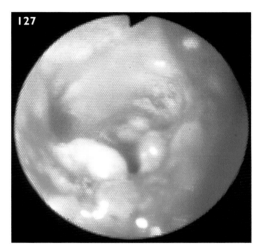

127 A rectal stricture endoscopically in Crohn's disease.

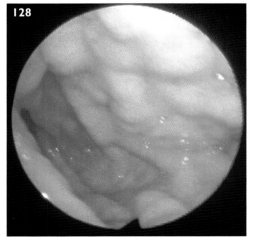

128 Nodular involvement of the duodenum in Crohn's disease seen at endoscopy.

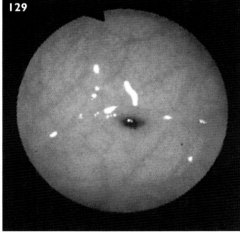

129 Opening of fistula track into the rectum.

Crohn's Disease

associated with abscess formation, surgical 'toilet' (probing under anaesthesia, incision of abscesses, conservative exploration to maintain drainage) may be necessary. In severe disease, proctectomy may be indicated.

Differential diagnosis
This varies depending on the major sites involved. Colonic Crohn's disease – ulcerative colitis, colonic or metastatic cancer, ischaemic colitis in the elderly. Ileocaecal Crohn's disease – tuberculosis, intestinal lymphoma. Chronic appendix abscess. Acute onset terminal ileal disease – *Yersinia* infection. Drugs (potassium chloride, non-steroidals) may cause gut ulceration.

Other differential diagnoses include other causes of malabsorption, i.e. coeliac disease, and gastrointestinal manifestations of immuno-deficiency.

Prognosis
Crohn's disease is currently regarded as 'disease for life'. The vast majority of patients have normal life expectancy, though some mortality due to severe disease and surgical complications occurs, particularly with complex fistulating disease. After surgery to remove disease, recurrence is usual after a mean of 5–10 years (**130**). In colonic Crohn's disease there is a small but definite increase in the risk of colonic cancer.

Complications
of Crohn's disease
Urinary problems in Crohn's disease include enterovesical fissure, or right hydronephrosis due to ileal obstruction.

Renal disease may occur if amyloidosis develops and in the presence of marked steatorrhoea, oxalate stones may form in the renal tract.

Gallbladder complications include gallstones (common, due to ileal disease and depletion of bile salt pool), and B_{12} deficiency (due to loss of B_{12} uptake sites which are limited to terminal ileum).

Management options
Medical
- Patient education; doctor/patient empathy (long-term follow-up is very important).
- In active inflammatory disease (high ESR, CRP), with knowledge of predominant site of disease: for small-intestinal disease: oral prednisolone – usually for several months –

some additional benefit from 5-amino-salicylic acid (5-ASA) (mesalazine): for colonic Crohn's disease – prednisolone (locally for distal disease, orally for pancolitis) and salazopyrine or mesalazine.
- Stop smoking.

Surgical Indications for surgery include failure to respond to medical treatment, chronic continuous disease, obstruction with fistulae, abscess. The most common indication for surgery is recurrent subacute obstruction due to fibrotic terminal ileal stenosis. About 70% of patients will come to surgery at some time.

Long-term treatment/other approaches
Recent evidence suggests that chances of relapse are reduced by taking 5-ASA long term. Some patients require long-term corticosteroids/immunosuppressants (i.e. azathioprine,6-mercaptopurine methotrexate) to control inflammation. Long-term corticosteroid therapy should preferably be avoided, and new 'poorly-absorbed' (and rapidly metabolised) steroids (e.g. budesonide) are now becoming available. Some dietary approaches (e.g. elemental diets) help to induce remission.

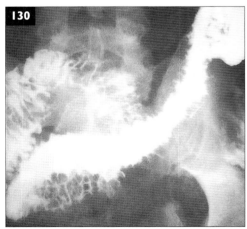

130 Recurrent ileal Crohn's disease in a patient with previous resections. A 'neo' terminal ileum lies in the normal position of the transverse colon, and is connected to the colon just before the splenic flexure.

Ileostomies

Definition
Ileostomies result from surgical operation, the procedure resulting in opening of the ileum through the anterior abdominal wall.

Characteristics
There are two types of ileostomy:
• Temporary ileostomies: performed as an interim stage when multistage colonic surgery is being performed.
• Permanent or 'spout ileostomies' (**131**): these are the most common type, and are used after removal of the colon (for ulcerative colitis or Crohn's disease). 'Continent' ileostomies (e.g. Koch's ileostomy) produce a pouch of ileum below the abdominal wall which is then drained intermittently via a catheter.

Permanent ileostomies are less common nowadays after total colectomy for ulcerative colitis or familial polyposis, as these conditions are now commonly treated by the creation of an ileoanal pouch.

Complications
• Local excoriation of skin and stoma.
• Subacute obstruction of distal ileum proximal to stoma.
• Excessive fluid loss and dehydration in hot weather.
• Urinary tract stone formation (urate stones) due to passage of concentrated acid urine, reflecting loss of alkali and fluid via ileostomy.
• Psychological problems. Support from fellow patients and stoma nurses is very helpful.

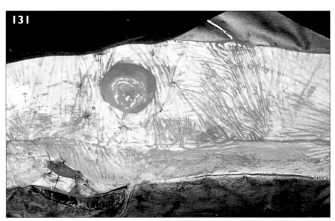

131 A spout ileostomy, formed in the right iliac fossa, seen just after completion by the surgeon.

Lymphoma of the Small Intestine

Definition
Malignant disease of lymphoid tissue of small intestine.

Epidemiology and aetiology
These are uncommon (but tumours of small intestine are overall uncommon). There are a number of distinct types:
- Primary small-intestinal lymphoma with no pre-existing cause. The lymphoma is of B-cell origin, occurs generally in the ileum, in males more often than females, and in young adults or elderly.
- Primary small-intestinal lymphoma with predisposing cause. These are of three sub-types:
  1. Lymphoma complicating adult coeliac disease – T-cell lymphoma in upper small intestine.
  2. Lymphoma complicating chronic infection 'Mediterranean lymphoma'. B-cells (IgA derived) in upper small intestine (**132–134**). There is a strong geographic incidence (Middle East, Southern Africa, in rural areas).
  3. Lymphoma complicating immuno-suppression – seen in HIV disease or in long-term immunosuppression.
- Secondary small-intestinal lymphoma – untreated or relapsing non-Hodgkin's lymphoma frequently affects the gut in its terminal stages.

Pathophysiology and aetiology
When a predisposing cause is identified, it appears that persistent antigenic challenge, e.g. gluten, multiple bacterial infection, leads to overexpression and development of a malignant clone of T- or B-cells. The pathophysiology reflects the nature of involvement, which may be diffuse (associated with wall thickening, loss of villous architecture, and obstruction of lymphatics) or consist of single or multiple deposits in the gut wall, leading to local complications. The spread is from the gut to the mesenteric lymph nodes, more distant lymph nodes and then systemically, including liver and spleen.

Clinical history
When there is no previous gut involvement, presentations are most often surgical emergencies (obstruction, bleeding or perforation, **135**). Diarrhoea, pain and malabsorption are less common presentations. Relapse in coeliac disease despite maintenance of a gluten-free diet is a classical presentation.

Examination
This is variable. Findings may include 'doughy' abdomen on palpation, and local masses. Hepatosplenomegaly and systemic lymphadenopathy are seen in advanced cases.

Laboratory and special examinations
Laboratory markers are often abnormal (high ESR, anaemia, hypoalbuminaemia) but non-specific. IgA and IgA heavy chains should be sought (see 'Special forms'). Anatomical studies – small-bowel enema may show irregular thickening of wall, areas of narrowing or dilatation, and diffuse or localised ulceration. Ultrasound and CT may show evidence of wall thickening and define lymphadenopathy.

Histology – mandatory for diagnosis – may require laparotomy/laparoscopy and full-thickness biopsy. One important aim of the investigation is to find the stage of disease.
- Stage I: One or more localised sites of gut.
- Stage II: Localised sites of gut plus regional lymph nodes.
- Stage III: Lymph nodes of both sides of the diaphragm with localised tumour of the gut.
- Stage IV: Diffuse or disseminated involvement of extralymphatic organs or tissues, with or without lymph node involvement.

Differential diagnosis
Crohn's disease and tuberculosis are the main differential diagnoses.

Prognosis
Prognosis is generally poor, reflecting the late stage at which the diagnosis is usually made.

Management
Surgery is often essential, as the presentation may be with surgical emergency, requiring local resection of obviously diseased tissue. Surgery may be curative, but is rarely so due to diffuse gastrointestinal involvement and late presentation. Therefore, systemic chemotherapy is more generally used.

Special forms
The rare Mediterranean lymphoma involves proliferation of IgA-producing B-cells. Diagnosis

Lymphoma of the Small Intestine

may be helped by the identification of abnormal free IgA heavy chain (part of the Ig molecule) in serum or other fluids. At an early stage this proliferation passes through an apparently benign form (immunoproliferative small-intestinal disease) in which antibiotic therapy, reducing antigenic challenge in the gut, may lead to reversal of the condition.

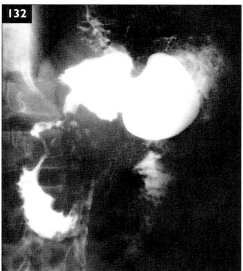

132 Extensive distortion of the first, second and third part of the duodenum in a patient with upper intestinal lymphoma (Mediterranean type).

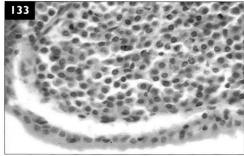

133 Jejunal biopsy in Mediterranean lymphoma showing infiltration with plasma cells (IgA-producing).

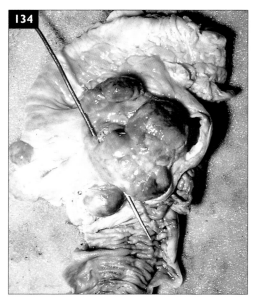

134 Nodular lymphoma (Mediterranean lymphoma) at autopsy.

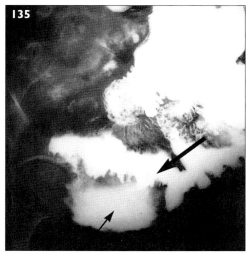

135 Lymphoma of the distal terminal ileum showing irregular thickening (thick arrow) of the walls, and a shapeless abscess cavity (thin arrow) just below as an indolent perforation has occurred.

Small-Intestinal Carcinoid Tumours

Definition
Tumours derived from enterochromaffin cells (subtype of endocrine cell) of the small intestine.

Aetiology and epidemiology
Carcinoid tumours are very common, but clinical problems from them rare, though possibly dramatic (**136**). Carcinoid tumours in the appendix (and rectum) are very common (up to 1% of the population), generally small and benign, and rarely symptomatic. Carcinoid tumours in the ileum, jejunum or duodenum may also be benign, but are likely to become malignant. A proportion of those that are malignant secrete hormones and other substances and give rise to the 'carcinoid syndrome'. Incidence is equal between sexes, and more common with advancing age, but can occur below the age of 30 years.

Pathology and pathophysiology
Primary tumours are smooth, submucosal nodules, generally asymptomatic, but with growth can ulcerate and bleed or lead to subacute obstruction. If they become malignant they infiltrate through the gut wall to the serosa and spread to the lymph nodes and liver (**137**). In addition, they can be associated with local thickening and fibrosis of the gut wall and mesentery (desmoplasia) as response to the tumour, making obstruction more likely (**138**). There are generally no systemic symptoms from release of hormones or other substances from primary tumour. If liver metastases occur, intermittent release into the circulation of substances such as serotonin can give rise to characteristics of carcinoid syndrome – flushing due to vasodilatation (see **136**), diarrhoea due to increased motility and gut secretion. In the long term, fibrosis of valves of the right side of the heart may lead to cardiac failure. In extreme cases, symptoms of pellagra may appear due to diversion of B vitamins to synthesise serotonin.

Clinical history
With primary tumour, symptoms are as for other primary tumours – obstruction, bleeding or incidentally found (e.g. at appendicectomy). With secondary tumour, presentation is either with hepatomegaly/pain (particularly with non-secreting tumours) or with symptoms of carcinoid syndrome. Secondary carcinoid tumours may be very slow growing, so survival with secondaries may be 10–20 years (mean 3–5 years). In carcinoid syndrome, episodes of flushing and diarrhoea occur, with sweating and in some patients also bronchoconstriction. With advanced disease, weight loss and cardiac failure may occur.

Physical examination
There is generally none at the primary stage. At the secondary stage, look for hepatomegaly (may be huge), peripheral oedema, thickening of skin, facial flushing (see **136**), conjunctivitis, permanent vasodilatation, tricuspid and pulmonary stenosis.

Laboratory and special examinations
For primary tumour, use small-bowel studies.
For secondary tumours, use ultrasound and CT to identify deposits in the liver and mesentery. A biopsy should be taken to confirm diagnosis. For suspected carcinoid syndrome, the 24-hour urinary excretion of 5-hydroxy-indole acetic acid (5-HIAA; a metabolite of serotonin) should be monitored, together with serum gut hormone.

Differential diagnosis
- At the primary stage, differentiate from other small-intestinal tumours.
- At the secondary stage, differentiate from other metastatic disease in the liver.

Carcinoid tumours can arise in sites other than the small intestine, and have varying tendencies to become malignant (rectum generally benign, colon commonly malignant), though neither of these gives rise to carcinoid syndrome. Bronchial adenomas may give rise to carcinoid syndrome, and may also become malignant.

Prognosis
This is variable. Prognosis for appendiceal carcinoid is very good, and surgery curative.

Management
For primary tumours without metastases, use a surgical approach.
In the case of carcinoid presenting with secondary deposits and no symptoms, management is difficult: chemotherapy or tumour debulking has not been demonstrated to prolong survival. For carcinoid syndrome, treatment depends on severity: control hormonal effects (ciproheptadine, somatostatin, surgical debulking, hepatic artery embolisation to devascularise tumours) or use chemotherapy (interferon, streptozotocin and 5-fluorouracil).

Small-Intestinal Carcinoid Tumours

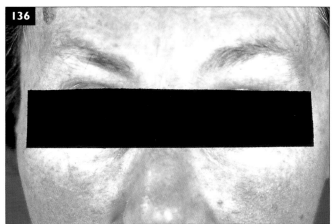

136 Face of a patient with carcinoid syndrome, showing flushing and telangiectasia.

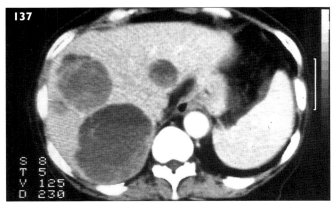

137 Large secondary deposits of carcinoid tumour in the liver on CT scan.

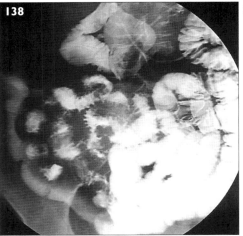

138 Extensive small-intestinal involvement with carcinoid primary in the terminal ileum. The distortion reflects fibrosis due to reaction in the tissues, not spread of the primary tumour itself.

Other Intestinal Tumours

BENIGN SMALL INTESTINAL TUMOURS
Benign tumours of the small intestine are rare. They may be derived from smooth muscle cells (leiomyoma, **139**), fat cells (lipoma), or nerve-elements (neuroma). They may present with obstruction or bleeding.

MALIGNANT SMALL INTESTINAL TUMOURS
Primary malignant tumours of the small intestine are much rarer than in either the colon or stomach. The main types are:
- Cancers.
- Carcinoid tumours (see below).
- Lymphomas (see previous section).

Small-intestinal cancers – these occur occasionally with predisposing cause (Crohn's disease, coeliac disease). Other cases occur in patients who carry a familial genetic predisposition (family cancer syndromes) who may have a strong family history of colonic, small-intestinal, breast and ovarian cancer.

Pathophysiology
Local deposits of tumour spread and infiltrate from the epithelium through the gut wall, and metastasise to the lymph nodes and liver.

Clinical history
Presentation is with pain, obstruction or bleeding. Because small-intestinal tumours are so rare, there is generally considerable delay in making the diagnosis. Some patients present with unexplained anaemia.

Physical examination
Only abnormal in advanced cases, with anaemia, local masses, subacute obstruction and hepatomegaly.

Laboratory and special examinations
Anaemia may be present. A high ESR indicates probable local or distant spread. No 'specific' tumour markers occur in the serum. A small-intestinal radiograph is not always diagnostic as tumours can be missed. Angiography, particularly in investigating 'chronic gastro-intestinal bleeding of unknown cause' may show vascular tumours. Laparotomy may be the final diagnostic test.

Prognosis
Poor, due to late stage presentation. The 5-year survival rate is less than 25%.

Treatment
Surgery is the main option. There is generally a poor response to adjuvant chemotherapy. Radiation is not helpful, as doses required would damage the remaining gut.

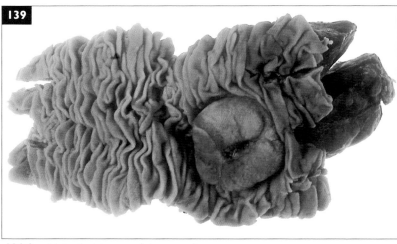

139 Small intestinal tumour (leiomyoma).

Intestinal Obstruction

Definition
The clinical picture is of obstruction of the intestinal lumen. This may be acute or subacute, and arise in small or large intestine. It may be incomplete or complete.

Epidemiology and aetiology
There are multiple causes in childhood – congenital stenosis, volvulus, 'Meconium ileus' in cystic fibrosis. In adults, the cause may be adhesions due to previous surgery. Tumours (140), hernias (141) and inflammatory processes (Crohn's disease in small intestine, diverticular disease and cancer in colon) are other causes.

Pathophysiology
In intestinal obstruction, secretion of fluid is induced proximally, leading to a clinical picture of distension and fluid loss into the gut and severe electrolyte disturbances.

Clinical history
The full-blown history of complete obstruction is colicky pain, distension, vomiting and constipation. More proximal obstruction causes vomiting earlier, more distal causes absolute constipation earlier.

Physical examination
Look for dehydration, abdominal distension and visible peristalsis (142). A rectal examination (low carcinoma/faecal impaction in the elderly) is mandatory.

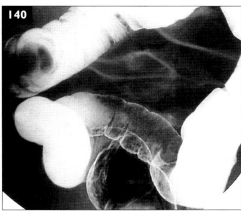

140 An uncommon cause of obstruction – intussuseption of a tumour, seen prolapsing into the transverse colon.

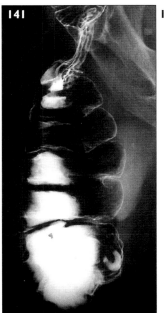

141 Remember hernias (particularly femoral hernias) as causes of obstruction. This is a barium X-ray showing prolapsing caecum into a right inguinal hernia.

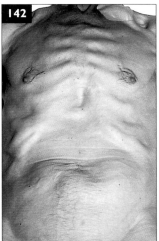

142 Small-intestinal obstruction – note the visible peristalsis.

Intestinal Obstruction

Investigations
General tests These include electrolytes (increased urea and creatinine), hypokalaemia and increased haemoglobin (representing dehydration). An initial blood screening should include cross-matching.

Specific tests A plain abdominal radiograph is most revealing (**143**). A supine radiograph is essential, an erect radiograph helpful. The presentation of dilated loops (fluid levels on erect film) often permits definition of the site of obstruction. A gastrointestinal follow-through with conventional radiograph (or CT) can help to define the site of obstruction (**144, 145**). In suspected low (colonic) obstruction, colonoscopy or barium enema may define the cause of obstruction from below, and barium enema should be performed before small-bowel radiograph.

Management
Resuscitation and restoration of fluid balance (nasogastric tube, intravenous fluids) vital. Allows time for further investigations. Unless symptoms resolve surgery will be indicated, but definition of cause helpful. Pseudo-obstruction should be excluded.

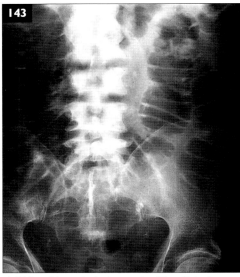

143 Small-intestinal obstruction. The dilated bowel is definitely small intestine, as the valvulae conniventes go from one side of the dilated bowel to the other. Note also the laminated gallstones in the right upper quadrant (and the large aortic aneurysm).

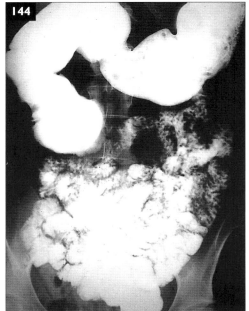

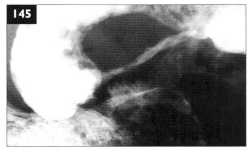

144 Duodenal obstruction – it is difficult to see where the stomach ends and the duodenum begins, but there is clearly obstruction in the duodenum.

145 The obstruction in **144** is due to a narrow segment of Crohn's disease in the 3rd part of duodenum, shown in this film.

Pseudo-Obstruction

Definition
The clinical picture is suggestive of obstruction in the absence of an obstruction to gut lumen (**146**). One particular form is 'paralytic ileus'; here there are distended fluid-filled, non-mobile loops of gut, most often seen after prolonged manipulation of the gut after surgery. Paralysis may also occur as a result of neglected small bowel obstruction.

Aetiology
Cases occur typically in:

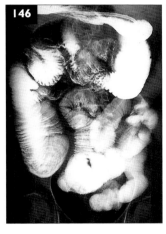

146 Pseudo-obstruction.

- Elderly, debilitated patients with severe illness (sepsis, circulatory failure).
- Patients with chronic disease affecting neural or neuromuscular supply of the gut (familial visceral neuropathy, familial visceral myopathy).
- Patients with retroperitoneal tumour.

The symptoms reflect a combination of loss of motility, and secondary bacterial overgrowth.

Clinical history
In severe illness, vomiting and distension may occur and differential diagnosis is that of organic bowel obstruction. In chronic pseudo-obstruction, patients present with distension, occasionally vomiting, intermittent pain and may have either constipation or diarrhoea.

Investigations
Initially, definition of patency of the entire gastrointestinal tract by contrast radiology, usually also showing slow transit. Biopsies may show abnormal muscle or absent nerves, but are often problematic. A full-thickness biopsy may be required. Conventional histology may be normal.

Prognosis
Progressive familial forms lead to malnutrition and require total parenteral nutrition. Repeated surgery is a hazard. Little can be done surgically, because postoperative ileus makes things worse. Because episodes are worse with bacterial overgrowth, intermittent antibiotic treatment may help.

Infections of the Small Intestine

VIRAL GASTROENTERITIS
This is an acute condition with nausea, vomiting and diarrhoea, generally self-limited (1–3 days). It is generally suspected rather than formally diagnosed. Causes are: rotavirus, calicivirus, astrovirus, Norwalk agent. The condition should be treated symptomatically. If diarrhoea is present, oral replacement of fluids and electrolytes can prevent dehydration without the use of intravenous fluids.

PROTOZOAL INFECTIONS
Giardiasis
This is a protozoal pathogen, transmitted by oral/faecal contamination. It contaminates the upper small intestine, and presents acutely with nausea, diarrhoea and weight loss. This may initiate a chronic malabsorptive state, particularly in immunodeficiency. Diagnosis is by analysis of duodenal fluid, duodenal biopsy, or (least efficient) cysts in the stool. Generally, responses to treatment with metronidazole are adequate, but repeat treatment may be necessary.

Cryptosporidiosis
This water-borne protozoan can cause acute self-limited diarrhoea in normals. The main clinical relevance is in the immunocompromised (notably AIDS), where it can cause protracted diarrhoea. It is identified histologically on light microscopy. Treatment with spiramycin is generally unsatisfactory.

Infections of the Small Intestine

BACTERIAL INFECTIONS
Salmonellosis
A wide variety of species of *Salmonella* give rise to acute enteritis. Systemic infections occur (with invasion) with *Salmonella typhi* and *S. paratyphi*, giving generalised fever, abdominal pain, often with constipation in the early stages and diarrhoea in late (second week). Invasion is via the terminal ileum lymphoid tissue. Perforation may occur.

Diagnosis Culture of blood, faeces and urine. Serology (Widal tests) are generally unreliable.

Treatment Treatment is with ampicillin, cipro-floxacin or chloramphenicol. Non-invasive *Salmonella* (e.g. *S. typhimurium*) gives enteritis with fever and diarrhoea, only occasionally with bleeding. Paradoxically, antibiotics may lead to prolongation of carriage. Diagnosis is performed on stool culture.

Campylobacter enteritides
A common cause of acute diarrhoea, with both small-intestinal and colonic colonisation. Presentation is with bloody diarrhoea and marked intestinal cramps and fever, often in small epidemics. Outbreaks frequently from the ingestion of poorly cooked chicken. The condition is only rarely invasive and is generally self-limited. Only treat with antibiotics if severe.

Cholera
Vibrio cholera is a bacterial, water-borne infection and is the cause of potentially devastating epidemics, particularly in the Third World and after civil or military upheaval. *Vibrio cholera* toxin binds to the surface of the enterocyte and induces secretion of sodium-rich fluid into small intestine, mainly by activation of cyclic AMP. The gut mucosa is not significantly inflamed. The result is many litres of fluid loss and diarrhoea, characteristically seen as the cholereic 'rice-water' stool.

Treatment Correction of fluid balance is the prime aim. Despite major activation of enterocyte secretion, the absorption capacity of cells is intact, so rather than intravenous therapy (which is often impracticable in cholera conditions) the use of 'cholera-replacement fluids' oral rehydration fluid recommended. These activate the glucose-dependent sodium pump. The typical constitution is sodium 90 mmol/l, glucose 111 mmol/l, potassium 20 mmol/l, citrate 10 mmol/l.

Antibiotics (tetracycline, trimethoprim–sulpha-methoxazole) are also indicated, but there is increasing resistance to these.

These oral rehydration fluids have been used extensively for treatment of all kinds of infectious diarrhoea, not only cholera, particularly in the Third World, and they represent a triumph of applied physiology.

TUBERCULOSIS ENTERITIS
This is a chronic infection caused by *Mycobacterium tuberculosis*. Both human and bovine strains can cause the disease. An atypical mycobacterium can cause infection, particularly in the immuno-suppressed. In the absence of immunosuppression, cases of tuberculous enteritis are rare in the West, except in immigrants. The condition is common in the developing world and may occur with or without pulmonary involvement. It occurs most often in the ileocaecal region (**147**) (differential diagnosis is Crohn's disease), but can also occur as diffuse upper small-intestinal disease (multiple strictures) or colonic disease.

Clinical manifestations
The condition presents with pain, diarrhoea, obstruction, or colonic bleeding, with variable weight loss. Ascites may be present (tuberculous peritonitis). Pulmonary tuberculosis is not always present.

Diagnosis and management
Contrast radiology shows an abnormal inflamed, irregular wall of the gut and strictures. A biopsy should be taken endoscopically if possible. Merely finding the mycobacterium in the stool is misleading (environmental mycobacteria may also be found), so specific identification is necessary. On suspicion, treatment is with conventional anti-tuberculous drugs.

CESTODES (TAPE WORMS)
Segmented flatworms
These include:
- *Taenia saginata* – beef tapeworm.
- *Taenia solium* – pork tapeworm.
- *Hymenolopsis nana* – dwarf tapeworm.
- *Diphyllobothrium latum* – fish tapeworm.

Ingestion by humans of infected meat or fish containing larval forms results in infestation of the small intestine. The worms stays anchored to the wall of the intestine by suckers or spikes sited on worm's head (or scolex). The worms are segmented, and eggs develop in the segments:

Infections of the Small Intestine

stool examination may reveal intact segments (proglottides) and eggs. The existence of adult worms is often asymptomatic, though obstruction may occur rarely. Pig tapeworm larvae may invade in humans, leading to cysticercosis, which affects the central nervous system and muscles. Niclosamide is the best treatment for intestinal infestation. Praziquantel treats both intestinal and systemic larval infestation.

Strongyloidiasis

Strongyloides worms colonise the upper gastrointestinal tract (**148,149**). In the immunosuppressed, or if there are anatomical abnormalities such as diverticulae, the worm can complete its whole reproductive cycle in the human tract. Hyperinfestation can lead to obstruction and bacterial septicaemia as worms carry bacteria into the body as they invade the mucosa. The infection commences by larvae penetrating the skin, trafficking to the lungs (causing pulmonary infiltration) and thence passing via the trachea to the oesophagus down to the duodenum where the adult worms develop. They may cause pain, diarrhoea, malabsorption and eosinophilia. Treatment is with thiabendazole, but eradication is difficult if there is anatomical abnormality or immunosuppression.

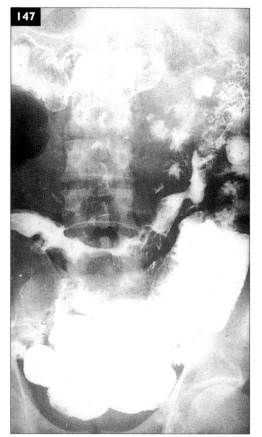

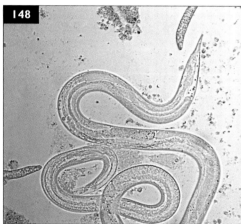

148 *Strongyloides stercoralis* – a worm colonising the upper small intestine.

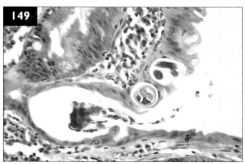

149 Infectious stronglyoides larvae, a cause of malabsorption in the immune suppressed.

147 Tuberculosis of the ileum and transverse colon. Note the dilatation of the small intestine proximal to obstruction in the terminal ileum area.

Vascular Disease of the Small Intestine

Definition

A variety of types of primary vascular pathology cause small-intestinal disease.

Arteriosclerotic disease This rarely causes gastrointestinal disturbance unless two of the three major arteries to the gut (coeliac, superior mesenteric artery and inferior mesenteric artery) are completely or partially occluded (150, 151). Normally, the rich collateral supply protects the small intestine, which is less susceptible to damage than the colon. Possible symptoms are:

- Mesenteric angina – pain after eating, leading to weight loss.
- Acute infarction (152) – precipitated by embolisation (atrial fibrillation, artificial valves, mural thrombosis after myocardial infarct), causes pain, paralytic ileus and may lead to perforation or localised peritonitis. In addition, low-flow states (e.g. heart failure) can cause paralytic ileus.

Venous thrombosis This may occur:

- In low-flow states.
- In hypercoagulable states, e.g. polycythaemia, deficiency of endogenous anticoagulants (protein C, protein S, antithrombin III, abnormal factor V).
- Secondary to severe dehydration.

The condition leads to pain and gastro-intestinal bleeding as a result of venous congestion. This may lead to portal venous obstruction, and the development of portal systemic collaterals, including oesophageal varices.

VASCULITIDES

Collagen vascular disorders can affect medium and small arteries of the small intestine (polyarteritis nodosa (153), Behçet's disease (154), lupus erythematosus) causing pain and bleeding, but rarely perforation and late complication of stricture. The colon can also be

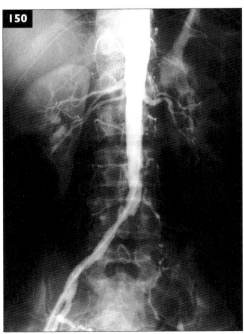

150 Anterior arteriogram showing renal arteries, but absence of left iliac, inferior mesenteric, and superior mesenteric arteries.

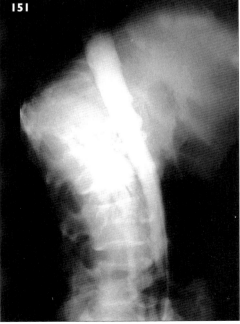

151 Lateral aortogram in a patient with mesenteric angina. There is an absence of the vessels which should normally be present – coeliac axis and superior mesenteric artery, on the anterior side of the aorta.

Vascular Disease of the Small Intestine

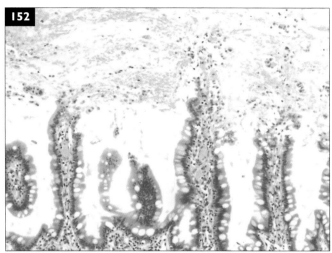

152 Histological specimen of small-intestinal mucosa showing severe ischaemia with exudation of pus from the surface.

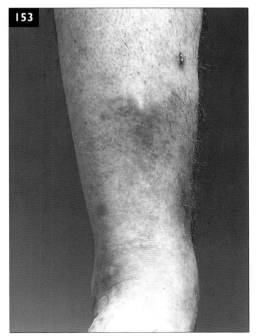

153 Systemic vasculitis with nodular involvement of the skin.

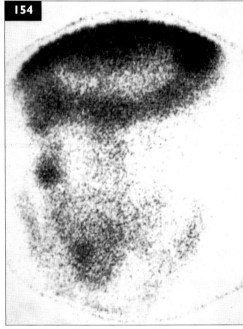

154 White cell scan showing diffuse patchy inflammation seen most prominently in the transverse colon in a patient with Behçet's disease (vasculitis).

Vascular Disease of the Small Intestine

involved (with a scenario as for colitis, **155**). The most common vasculitis is Henoch–Schönlein purpura – a response to exogenous antigens (e.g. *Streptococcus*, some foods) which gives a triad of:
- Skin rash (**156**).
- Acute glomerulonephritis (red cell casts in urine, increase in blood pressure, oedema.
- Gastrointestinal involvement – terminal ileum inflammation with pain (often due to intussusception) and bleeding (**157**).

Most cases of Henoch–Schönlein purpura resolve spontaneously, although on occasion, corticosteroids may be indicated. A minority of patients progress to renal failure.

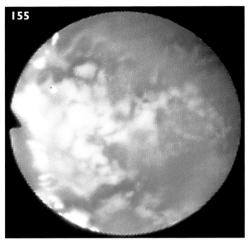

155 Endoscopic appearance of colonic mucosa in acute vasculitis.

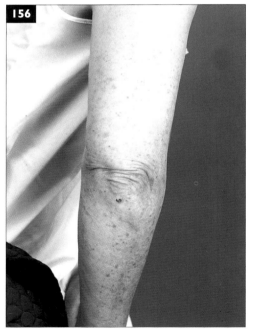

156 Vasculitis area on the extensor surfaces in Henoch–Schönlein purpura.

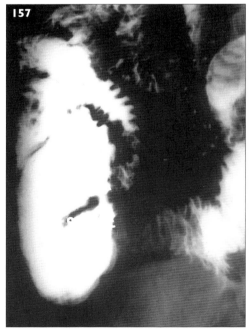

157 Barium follow-through of terminal ileum showing oedematous terminal ileum (Henoch–Schönlein purpura).

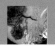

Chapter Six

Pancreas

Symptomatically it may be difficult to discover that the pancreas is abnormal

Acute pancreatitis is a major medical emergency

Chronic pancreatitis may be difficult to diagnose

Pancreatic cancer often presents late, yet early diagnosis is vital if there is to be a chance of cure

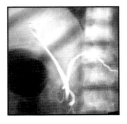
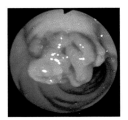
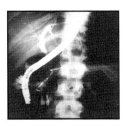
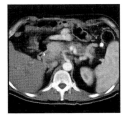

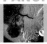

Anatomy

The pancreas lies transversely across the abdomen retroperitoneally. Its ductal system reflects its embryonic origin and occasionally there may be two openings of pancreatic ducts into the duodenum (the ampulla of Vater, and accessory ampulla) (**158**). The pancreatic head, body and tail drain through the pancreatic duct into the duodenum.

Histology
The pancreatic acini, which secrete pancreatic enzymes, drain into the pancreatic ductules and then the duct. The islets of Langerhans are 'neuroendocrine tissues' which are scattered throughout the pancreatic parenchyma.

Investigations
These include:
- Plain radiograph: this may show pancreatic calcification.
- Ultrasound, CT and MRI scans: these may show enlargement or irregularity of the pancreas, surrounding inflammation, and the presence of cysts, pseudocysts, mass lesions or dilatation of ducts. Ultrasound may be difficult due to overlying gas.
- Barium radiograph: this is of little use unless the second and third parts of the duodenum are distorted by inflammation or tumour.
- Endoscopic retrograde cholangiopancreato-graphy (ERCP) (**159**): this is now the main anatomical investigation; it should show the normal duct, duct distortion or dilatation in chronic pancreatitis, obstruction, or tumour mass.
- Direct percutaneous fine needle aspiration of masses: this can be performed under ultrasound or CT guidance.

Functional tests These rely on evidence of pancreatic exocrine function.

Tube tests These include the Lundh test meal and secretin test. They require duodenal intubation and recovery of pancreatic juice after a test meal, or injection of the hormone, secretin, to stimulate pancreatic secretion. Classical results in chronic pancreatitis show a normal volume of dilute pancreatic juice, i.e. low bicarbonate secretion, low protein. In cancer of the pancreas, results show a small volume of normal pancreatic juice (though these groups often overlap). These tests are now rarely used.

Tubeless tests Here, a substrate given by mouth is broken down by active pancreatic enzyme: e.g. para-aminobenzoic acid (PABA) test uses PABA bound to fluorescein, given by mouth. If digested normally, the fluorescein is split off and secreted in the urine. Excretion >30% is taken as normal.

Anatomy

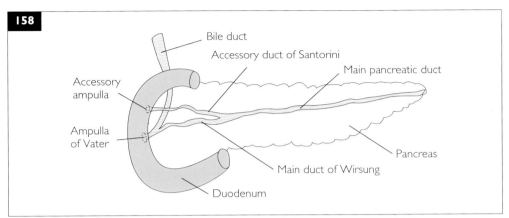

158 The pancreatic gland drains through two ducts, the main duct
(Wirsung) through the ampulla of Vater, joining the bile ducts;
the minor duct (Santorini) through an accessory ampulla
There are a variety of anatomical aberrations.

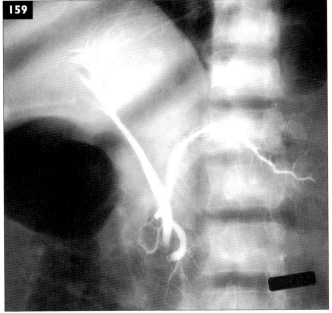

159 Normal pancreatic duct and biliary duct shown at ERCP.

Acute Pancreatitis

Definition
A clinical syndrome characterised by acute inflammation of the pancreas. Abdominal pain and abnormal serum pancreatic enzyme levels are typical.

Epidemiology and aetiology
All populations are affected, though with significant variability related to the prevalence of predisposing causes. Gallstones, particularly in the common bile duct, constitute the single largest cause (30–85%), increasing the risk by 12- to 35-fold. Alcohol is implicated in ~5% of cases of acute pancreatitis, but note that in chronic alcoholics acute-on-chronic pancreatitis is a common problem. Other causes include trauma, drugs (e.g. azathioprine, pentamidine or thiazide diuretics), infectious agents (e.g. mumps, HIV) hyperlipidaemia (triglycerides usually >500 mg/dl) and hypercalcaemia. ERCP causes pancreatitis rarely (0.4–1.2%).

Pathophysiology
The precise mechanisms are complex. Pancreatic ductal obstruction is involved. Trypsinogen activation within the pancreatic acinar cells, impaired secretion of enzymes, and cell auto-digestion all occur. These lead to interstitial oedema, inflammatory cell infiltration, tissue necrosis, and may lead on to damage to contiguous or distant organs and multi-organ failure.

Clinical history
Abdominal pain is most frequent, usually in the epigastric or umbilical region, with radiation to the back. Classically, pain is relieved by sitting and leaning forward, although this is uncommon. The pain may be extremely severe, may not peak for several hours, and is usually not relieved by vomiting. Nausea and vomiting are generally present. In advanced or severe pancreatitis, confusion, coma or respiratory failure may occur.

Physical examination
Typical symptoms are tachycardia, hypotension and fever. High-grade fever may be encountered with cholangitis or severe tissue necrosis. Jaundice is usually absent. Severe jaundice may indicate biliary obstruction or liver disease. Shock may be present. Abdominal tenderness, rigidity and sluggish or absent bowel sounds may be found. Retroperitoneal haemorrhage may discolour the skin around the umbilicus or flanks (Grey Turner's sign).

Rarely, subcutaneous fat necrosis by circulating pancreatic enzymes may manifest with painful nodules (panniculitis).

Laboratory and special examinations
Biochemical tests There is increased serum amylase level (specificity ~95% when serum amylase is >3-fold that of normal subjects). Serum lipase (more specific) is the best enzyme marker. Serum amylase and lipase levels rise simultaneously early; serum amylase may return to normal within 24 hours, whereas serum lipase remains elevated for several days. Enzyme isoforms, such as L2 pancreatic lipase or pancreatic amylase enhance specificity. The renal clearance of amylase may be increased by tubular dysfunction and is not diagnostic. Acute phase reactants, such as neutrophil elastase, interleukin-6 or C-reactive protein are non-specific. Serum bilirubin, aspartate aminotransferase (AST), alanine aminotransferase (ALT) and alkaline phosphatase help evaluate coexisting biliary disease.

Radiology Use plain radiographs of the chest and abdomen for detecting pleural effusion, 'sentinel loop' (160) or a perforation. Use abdominal ultrasound for gallstones or gallbladder 'sludge', although intestinal gas or obesity often limit pancreatic imaging. CT is often necessary and demonstrates necrosis and/or extrapancreatic fluid collection. ERCP is indicated for ductal trauma or obstruction, e.g. by gallstones and parasites.

Differential diagnosis
Other causes of acute abdomen
These include acute cholecystitis, perforated peptic ulcer, acute intestinal obstruction, nephrolithiasis, ruptured aneurysm of abdominal aorta, ruptured liver abscess or tumour, acute salpingo-oophoritis, etc.

Disease of other organs These include lobar pneumonia, pleural disease, and CNS disease, e.g. subarachnoid haemorrhage when confusion or coma are predominant.

Abnormal serum amylase In addition to acute pancreatitis, this indicates renal disease, salivary gland disease, and other acute abdominal events including perforation of a duodenal ulcer. Macroamylasaemia in association with another cause for abdominal pain may be particularly confusing. In macroamylasaemia, large complexes of amylase and immunoglobulins, or amylase polymers,

Acute Pancreatitis

cannot be cleared by renal tubules and circulate in the blood. The diagnosis is established by demonstrating low renal amylase clearance and by gel filtration to demonstrate macroamylase.

Prognosis
The prognosis is highly variable, ranging from uneventful recovery to multiple complications, protracted course and death.

The Ranson or Glasgow criteria utilise age, white blood cell count (WBC), lactate dehydrogenase (LDH), glucose, AST, albumin, calcium, arterial pO_2, and blood urea, at admission and within 48 hours to assign prognosis.

The Acute Physiology and Chronic Health Evaluation (APACHE) III criteria use 14 routinely measured parameters and can be more quickly obtained.

The CT Severity Index is based upon pancreatic enlargement, extent of inflammation, peripancreatic fluid collection and degree of tissue necrosis, and correlates with observations at surgery, as well as the Ranson criteria.

Early complications include fluid and electrolyte imbalances, gastrointestinal haemorrhage, shock, adult respiratory distress syndrome, and renal failure. Late complications include pancreatic ascites, pancreatic abscess, pseudocyst or fistula (see 'Complications of pancreatitis', p. 122).

Management
The mainstays are supportive care and prevention of complications. No curative treatments are available. Replacement of fluid and electrolyte deficits and correction of metabolic abnormalities are important. Nasogastric aspiration is of unproven value except when ileus exists. Protein intake is generally restricted and proteins are gradually reintroduced. A period of intravenous hyperalimentation may be beneficial. Antibiotics, endoscopic papillotomy and other measures may be necessary for complications. Emergency pancreatic surgery or inhibitors of pancreatic secretion are not generally indicated, although in severe disease with complications, such as abscesses or extensive pancreatic necrosis, surgery may be required.

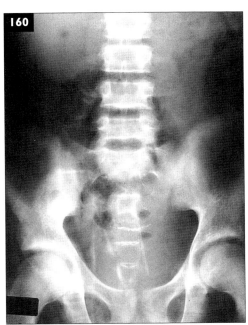

160 Acute pancreatitis – note the sentinel loop of jejunum adjacent to the pancreas.

Chronic Pancreatitis

Definition
Progressive and permanent pancreatic damage resulting in tissue loss, morphologic change and/or abnormal function. Several classifications have been proposed based upon aetiology, clinical presentation and morphological change, such as pancreatic fibrosis, obstruction and calcification.

Epidemiology and aetiology
Prevalence is ill-defined, and varies widely among populations. One Western survey of the annual incidence of chronic pancreatitis was 8/100 000 and prevalence 26/100 000. Prolonged alcohol intake is the most frequent cause (~70%). Idiopathic pancreatitis (10–40%) may present in younger (second decade) or older (sixth decade) age groups. Other causes (<10%) include tropical pancreatitis, hereditary pancreatitis, hyperparathyroidism, mechanical obstruction of the main pancreatic duct and trauma.

Pathophysiology
The characteristic features are inflammatory changes, progressive atrophy, starting in acinar tissue followed by pancreatic islets, and fibrosis. The pancreatic ducts are dilated, particularly in the 'obstructive' form. The 'lithogenic' type is marked by intraductal plugs or stones and chronic calcification of the pancreas. There is altered secretion of pancreatic enzymes, which promotes the autodigestion of tissues. An increased viscosity of pancreatic juice aids plug formation, ductal obstruction and fibrosis. Pain is probably related to intrapancreatic distension and release of local neurotransmitters.

Clinical history
Abdominal pain is most common. The pain is epigastric, dull and constant, radiates to the back, worsened by food, and occurs in bouts lasting several days or weeks interspersed with pain-free intervals. Pain may continue unchanged, disappear, or decrease with the onset of pancreatic calcification or steatorrhoea. The latter occurs when enzyme secretion is reduced by >90%, usually after 10–20 years. Diabetes mellitus may develop between 5–18 years after the onset of pancreatitis. In 15% of cases, chronic pancreatitis may be painless. Other symptoms include nausea, vomiting, anorexia, weight loss due to fear of pain upon eating or malabsorption, jaundice, ascites or pleural effusion.

Physical examination
Look for cachexia, or evidence of weight loss, epigastric tenderness, occasionally abdominal distension in the setting of complications, such as pseudocyst.

Laboratory and special examinations
Serum amylase levels are usually normal. In severe disease, serum pancreatic polypeptide levels may rise less in response to a protein test-meal or intravenous secretin. Tests of exocrine pancreatic function are of limited value because duodenal intubation is necessary for sampling pancreatic juice, results may vary from laboratory to laboratory, and unequivocal abnormalities require extensive disease. The characteristic pattern is subnormal pancreatic enzyme and bicarbonate content of the pancreatic juice.

Many 'indirect' tests of pancreatic insufficiency, such as faecal chymotrypsin, dual Schilling test, or ^{14}C-olein absorption suffer from inadequate sensitivity and specificity. Some tubeless tests which depend on urinary recovery of a marker such as fluorescein, which needs to be split from a complex by pancreatic enzymes after ingestion, may be helpful but they depend on adequate urine collection.

Radiology Plain radiograph of the abdomen may show diffuse, speckled calcification (30–40%) (161). In this case, no further testing is necessary.

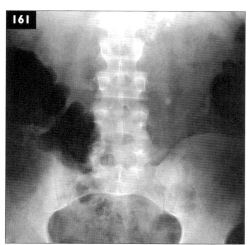

161 Plain abdominal X-ray showing calcification in the pancreas (chronic pancreatitis).

Chronic Pancreatitis

Ultrasound and CT (sensitivity and specificity ~90%) may show a small pancreas with altered texture, dilated main pancreatic duct (>4 mm), oedema, cavities, calcification and pseudocysts. ERCP is the 'gold standard' (specificity up to 100%) (**162–165**) and disease may be graded

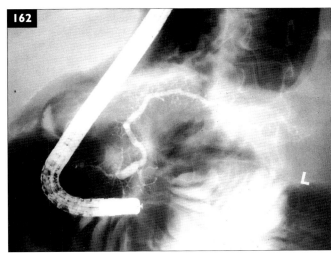

162 Minor irregularities of the ducts in a patient with chronic pancreatitis of the pancreatic duct.

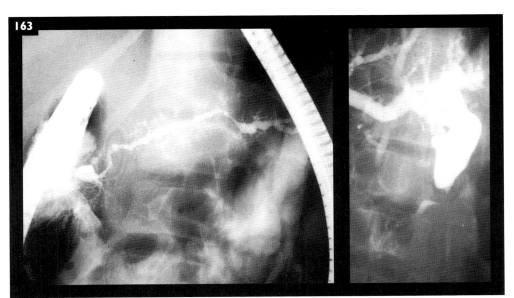

163 ECRP in a patient with chronic pancreatitis (in the left-hand side there are only minor changes in the pancreatic duct; on the right-hand side, the hardened pancreatic head has caused obstruction to the common bile duct and intrahepatic tree).

Chronic Pancreatitis

into minimal (minor duct dilatation, intraductal calculi), moderate (dilated, tortuous or stenotic main pancreatic duct) or advanced (addition of cystic changes) pancreatitis.

Differential diagnosis
Differentiate from pancreatic carcinoma, acid peptic disease, biliary disease and occult malignancy.

Prognosis
Chronic pancreatitis is an indolent disorder with periodic symptomatic exacerbations, leading over a number of years to total organ failure. There is a greater risk of pancreatic carcinoma. Obstructive biliary complications or other complications (see below) increase morbidity. Chronic alcoholism also predisposes to other diseases, such as infectious complications. Addiction to narcotic analgesics may pose difficulties.

Management
The mainstays are pain relief and improved nutritional status. Abstinence from alcohol is helpful in the long term, but does not reverse disease. Non-narcotic analgesics are used where possible, although opiates are usually necessary. Oral replacement of pancreatic enzymes diminishes pancreatic stimulation, intraductal pressure, pain and malabsorption. Simultaneous gastric acid suppression and use of enteric-coated formulations improve the efficacy of enzyme replacement. Percutaneous injection of alcohol into the celiac ganglion may help refractory pain, although the benefit lasts for only 3–6 months. Endoscopic therapy for papillary stenosis, stricture or stone, including by sphincterotomy, stenting or balloon dilatation may help. Surgery may be necessary for localised ductal obstruction, and partial pancreatic resection, as well as pancreatico-jejunostomy are occasionally performed.

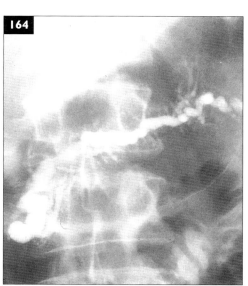

164 Severe chronic pancreatitis seen after ERCP (endoscope removed); there is a widened ectatic tortuous pancreatic duct.

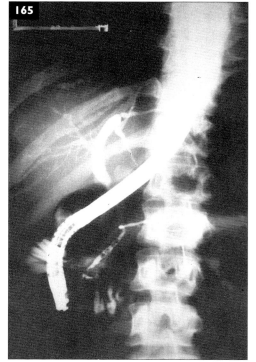

165 ERCP showing the pancreatic duct and the presence of intraductal calculi. The biliary tract is also demonstrated.

Inherited Pancreatic Disorders

CYSTIC FIBROSIS (CF)
The commonest inherited pancreatic disorder characterised by abnormally viscid exocrine secretions due to defective activation of a cAMP-dependent chloride channel.

Epidemiology and aetiology
An autosomally recessive disorder, CF is transmitted in 1 per 2500 live Caucasian births. The gene frequency approaches 5% in North Europeans. CF is also prevalent in southern Europe, Ashkenazi Jews and African Americans. Heterozygote carriers are asymptomatic. Abnormality of CF gene affects cystic fibrosis transmembrane conductance regulator (CFTR) (a 3-base-pair DNA deletion in codon 508 of exon 10). Normally, the cAMP-dependent CFTR in apical cell membranes of epithelial or duct cells allows flow of chloride and bicarbonate, which leads to net fluid secretion and alkalinisation. In CF, there is defective dilution and alkalinisation of exocrine secretions, including those in pancreatic ducts, bile ducts, bronchial epithelium and sweat glands.

Pathophysiology
There is increased viscosity of exocrine secretions and increased electrolyte concentrations in sweat and saliva. The consequences include intrauterine growth retardation, impaired foetal development, meconium ileus (obstruction of neonatal gut), recurrent respiratory infection, bronchiectasis, chronic obstructive pulmonary disease, focal biliary cirrhosis, pancreatic exocrine insufficiency and male genital tract lesions in the ductal systems. The pancreas is small, irregular and cystic with eosinophilic duct concretions. Dilatation of ducts, enzyme leaks and cycles of autodigestion lead to fat, fibrosis and cystic changes, eventually impairing pancreatic islet function. Pancreatic insufficiency develops in >80% of patients, with gallbladder disease in 50% and gallstones in 12%.

Clinical history
Diarrhoea and steatorrhoea are the most common gastroenterological findings.

Physical examination
No specific abdominal abnormalities may be detected. Cholestasis may be associated with mild to moderate hepatomegaly. Biliary cirrhosis may develop.

Laboratory and special examinations
The diagnosis is made by increased Na^+ and Cl^- concentrations, >77 mmol/l and >74 mmol/l, respectively. Chromosomal analysis using molecular genetic methods can also be done in appropriate laboratories. Steatorrhoea may be demonstrated by analysis of stool fat. Imaging modalities of ultrasound, CT and ERCP are employed as discussed above.

Differential diagnosis
Differentiate from other causes of pancreatic insufficiency.

Prognosis
With improving attention to respiratory complications, the median survival has increased to 29 years. Some patients survive to the fifth decade. The most critical factors are prevention of dehydration and infectious repiratory events.

Management
Pancreatic insufficiency is managed in the standard fashion. The goals are to relieve pain and steatorrhoea. Efforts towards effective gene therapy are aimed at expressing normal copies of the CFTR gene in affected epithelia.

SCHWACHMAN'S SYNDROME
This is the second most common pancreatic disorder in children. It is an autosomal recessive condition, affecting 1 in 20 000 births. In addition to pancreatic exocrine insufficiency, abnormalities include haematological abnormalities (cyclical neutropenia, anaemia, thrombocytopenia or pancytopenia), bone disorders (metaphyseal dysostosis, short stature), eczema, diabetes mellitus and Hirschsprung's disease. Failure to thrive and steatorrhoea occur. The pancreas is small and fatty. Infection is an important cause of mortality. Treatment is mainly supportive. Symptoms may spontaneously improve with age in some patients.

HEREDITARY PANCREATITIS
A familial syndrome characterised by recurrent pancreatitis from early childhood and throughout life. Autosomal dominant, with a high penetrance (~80%). The disorder accounts for 5–10% of chronic pancreatitis cases. The deficiency of a pancreatic lithoprotein which normally inhibits pancreatic stone formation is believed to be involved. The mean age of onset is 10 years. The clinical presentation is characterised by prolonged attacks of pain, large calculi in major pancreatic ducts, frequent pancreatic calcification and an increased incidence of pancreatic adenocarcinoma.

Complications of Pancreatitis

The onset may be acute or insidious. Adjacent organs may be affected by the inflammatory process, e.g. sympathetic pleural effusions. The following are more specific complications which may occur in both acute and chronic pancreatitis.

PSEUDOCYST
This involves collection of pancreatic juice enclosed by fibrous tissue within or without the pancreas, but in any case beyond the normal pancreatic duct system. Pseudocysts develop in 25% of patients with chronic pancreatitis and in 10% with acute pancreatitis. They are more common in the body than the head or tail of the pancreas.

Symptoms
Include pain, early satiety or gastric outlet obstruction. Pancreatic pseudocysts may rupture, bleed, produce ascites, obstruct bile flow, compress the inferior vena cava, erode into the mediastinum or become infected. Chronic pseudocysts cause fewer complications. Pseudocysts >6 cm in size do not resolve spontaneously.

Diagnosis
Diagnosis may require ultrasound, CT(**166**) or ERCP, although infection can be introduced at ERCP (**167**).

Treatment
Pseudocysts are treated by CT-guided percutaneous drainage (90% success), by endoscopic drainage into the stomach or by surgical excision and internal or external drainage.

PANCREATIC INFECTION
Significant necrosis, as in acute pancreatitis, predisposes to infection. Recurrence of pain, fever, leucocytosis or bacteraemia within 1–2 weeks of acute pancreatitis is often a presenting manifestation. Indolent abscesses may present after several weeks.

Diagnosis requires CT-guided needle aspiration and Gram stain and culture.

Treatment requires prompt institution of broad-spectrum antibiotics; surgical debridement may also be necessary.

Mortality ranges from 15–100%, depending upon promptness in diagnosis, aggressive treatment, identification of infectious organisms and antibiotic susceptibility, as well as host factors.

SPLENIC VEIN THROMBOSIS
In coursing along the posterior surface of the pancreas, the splenic vein can be thrombosed due to peripancreatic oedema, inflammation or seepage. Splenic vein thrombosis is five times more common in chronic compared with acute pancreatitis. The condition causes extrahepatic portal hypertension, splenomegaly and gastric varices.

Diagnosis is by Doppler ultrasound or celiac angiography. Splenectomy cures gastric varices.

PANCREATIC ASCITES
Pancreatic secretions may enter the peritoneal cavity during acute, as well as chronic, pancreatitis. The ascites is characterised by elevated total protein, serum albumin and pancreatic enzyme content. Coexisting pseudocysts are found in 60% of cases. Pancreatic ascites may develop in 15% of patients with chronic pancreatitis.

Most patients require surgery. ERCP may help to localise the pancreatic leak.

PANCREATIC FISTULA
External fistulae are rare. Most are internal and occur after drainage or rupture of a pseudocyst, trauma and surgery. The draining fluid is enriched in amylase. ERCP or a fistulogram help make the diagnosis. Management is usually conservative. Stenting of the duct, or use of the long-acting somatostatin analogue, octreotide, to suppress pancreatic secretion or surgery may be necessary.

Complications of Pancreatitis

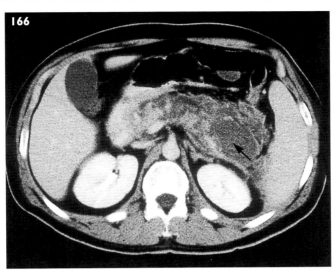

166 CT scan showing a large pseudocyst (arrowed) in a swollen, oedematous pancreas.

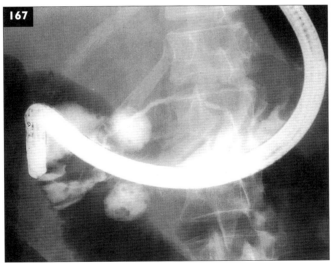

167 In addition to the pancreatic duct, there are cysts shown in connection with the duct.

Endocrine Pancreatic Tumours

Definition
Tumours arising from the neuroendocrine system and sharing characteristics of amine precursor uptake and decarboxylation (APUDomas).

Epidemiology and aetiology
These are uncommon tumours, with a prevalence estimated at <10 cases per million population. Gastrinomas and insulinomas are the most frequent (1–3 cases/million/year) compared with all other tumour types (<0.2 cases/ million/year), including glucagonoma, somatostatinoma, vasoactive intestinal peptide (VIP)-oma, growth hormone-releasing factor (GRF)-oma and pancreatic polypeptide (PP)-oma. Non-functioning endocrine tumours are more frequent (1% of all tumours found at autopsy, 36% of pancreatic endocrine tumours). Tumours may be sporadic or part of the multiple endocrine neoplasia (MEN) I syndrome, an autosomal dominant disorder affecting chromosome 11 with parathyroid, pancreas and pituitary tumours.

Pathophysiology and pathology
Typically, monotonous sheets of small, round cells with uniform nuclei and cytoplasm. Mitotic figures are few, consistent with their slow-growing nature. Electron microscopy shows granules containing peptide hormones and other characteristic substances (e.g. amines, neurone-specific enolase, chromogranin). Tumours may produce more than one hormone. Histological typing does not predict the tumour growth pattern. The diagnosis of malignancy requires evidence for invasion of adjacent organs, lymph nodes, liver (**168**) or blood vessels. Only 5–10% of insulinomas are malignant, whereas 50–90% of other tumour types are malignant. The size of the tumours correlates with the malignancy potential. Similar endocrine tumours may be found in lungs, jejunum, duodenum or elsewhere.

History and physical findings
Manifestations depend upon the specific peptide produced by the tumours:
- Gastrinoma. Typically, recurrent duodenal ulceration, diarrhoea and hypergastrinaemia constitutes the Zollinger–Ellison syndrome.
- Insulinoma. Excess insulin release produces recurrent hypoglycaemia, weight gain in a subconscious effort to avoid hypoglycaemia, psychiatric manifestations, palpitations, dizziness and sweating.
- VIPOMA. Watery secretory diarrhoea, hypokalaemia, achlorhydria (WDHA syndrome; Verner–Morrison syndrome) and occasionally hyperglycaemia, hypercalcaemia or flushing.
- Glucagonoma (**169**). Necrolytic migratory erythema (annular erythema affecting buttocks, groin, perineum or thighs, superficial bullae, erosions with crusting and hyperpigmentation), cheilitis, alopecia and nail dystrophy. Also, glucose intolerance, anaemia, weight loss, diarrhoea, hypoaminoacidaemia, thromboembolism, occasionally psychiatric manifestations and elevated erythrocyte sedimentation rate.
- Somatostatinoma. Hyperglycaemia, gallbladder disease, diarrhoea or steatorrhoea, hypochlorhydria and weight loss.
- GRFOMA. Acromegaly is characteristic but may not be seen in all patients. Abdominal complaints related to hepatic metastases may be prominent. Often associated with Zollinger–Ellison syndrome or MEN I.
- PPOMA and non-functioning tumours. No specific symptoms related to peptide release. Cachexia, abdominal pain, hepatomegaly, gastrointestinal hypermotility, decreased gastric acid production or exocrine pancreatic secretion.
- Other tumours. Cushing's syndrome due to corticotrophin release; hypercalcaemia due to increased parathormone production, etc.

Laboratory and special examinations
Diagnosis requires gut hormone assays to identify increased plasma levels of specific peptides, functional studies to demonstrate physiological consequences of peptide excess and imaging studies to demonstrate tumour. Various modalities include ultrasound (sensitivity 10–40%), CT (sensitivity 17–40%), endoscopic ultrasound (sensitivity >80%), selective coeliac angiography (sensitivity 35–90%) and multiple venous sampling for peptide assays, MRI (25–100% sensitivity) and intraoperative ultrasound (sensitivity >90%).

Differential diagnosis
Endocrine tumours simulate many common disorders and a reasoned approach is essential.

Prognosis
The 5- to 10-year survival rates are >90% when either no tumour is found (and by implication is

Endocrine Pancreatic Tumours

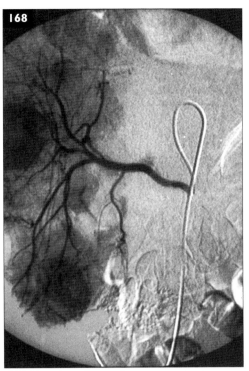

168 Hepatic angiogram in a neuroendocrine tumour of the liver showing massive hypervascular deposits.

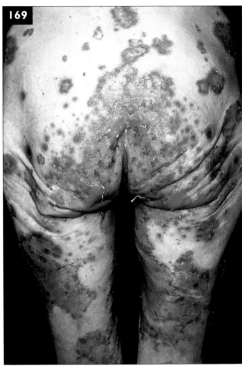

169 The characteristic rash in a patient with a glucagonoma.

very small), or tumour can be completely resected at surgery; rates are 15–75% with incomplete tumour resection or recurrent tumour; and 20–75% with unresectable tumours.

Management
Medial management may require the use of either specific peptide antagonists or symptomatic treatments to control metabolic abnormalities. Somatostatin analogues are useful in treating manifestations of VIPOMA, as well as glucagonoma. Proton pump inhibitors at high dose or H_2 antagonists are essential in gastrinoma (Zollinger–Ellison syndrome) to prevent gastroduodenal acid-mediated damage. Surgical outcomes improve with greater experience in tertiary referral centres. Chemotherapy used for metastatic endocrine tumours is commonly streptozotocin, 5-fluorouracil, doxorubicin or interferons. Debulking surgery may be undertaken. Symptomatic hepatic metastases may be treated by hepatic artery embolisation. Orthotopic liver transplantation may improve survival in selected patients.

Cancer of the Exocrine Pancreas

Definition
Primary adenocarcinoma originating in pancreatic cells (excluding endocrine elements).

Epidemiology and aetiology
Tumours may originate from pancreatic ducts (88%), acinar cells (1%), connective tissue (0.6%), mixed cell-type (0.2%) and of uncertain or unclassified histogenesis (9%). The incidence of pancreatic adenocarcinoma (ductal origin) has risen to 11–12/100 000 of the population. The most affected age group is between 60–80 years (80%) and the disease is uncommon in those aged under 40 years. The prevalence is greater in chronic pancreatitis (>9-fold increase), diabetics (2–3-fold increase), chronic smokers (~2-fold increase), urban populations, and after exposure to industrial carcinogens.

Pathophysiology and pathology
The precise role of specific risk factors is unknown. There are well-differentiated, duct-like glands embedded in a dense matrix of fibrous tissue. The majority of pancreatic adenocarcinomas produce mucin (75%) and are located in the head of the pancreas. The tumours frequently extend to the retroperitoneum or invade adjacent organs, such as stomach, duodenum or gallbladder. Distant metastases are more frequently noted, with tumours arising in the body or tail of the pancreas.

Clinical history
Symptoms depend upon the location of the tumour. Lesions affecting the ampulla of Vater present early with obstructive jaundice (170). Tumours in the head of the pancreas may present with biliary (171) or more rarely duodenal obstruction. Tumours arising in the body and tail (172) tend to be 'silent' and therefore larger when they eventually become symptomatic. Poorly localised abdominal pain, anorexia, fatigue and weight loss are frequent. Neuropsychiatric manifestations, including depression and emotional lability may be noted. Pruritus may be persistent.

Physical examination
Hepatomegaly and jaundice are noted in 80% of cases, palpable gallbladder in 30% with carcinoma of the head of the pancreas, and abdominal mass, ascites and oedema in 20%.

Laboratory and special examinations
Serum alkaline phosphatase, bilirubin or blood sugar may be elevated. Plain radiograph of the abdomen may show calcification of chronic pancreatitis. Pancreatic adenocarcinoma itself almost never calcifies. 'Sunburst' calcification is characteristic of benign cystadenoma. A cavernous lymphangioma of pancreas may also calcify. Circulating antigens, including carcinoembryonic antigen, CA 19-9 and CA 125, have no diagnostic role by themselves, because they may be elevated in inflammatory disease.

Radiology
Imaging studies are most helpful. Ultrasound and CT (173) (sensitivity and specificity 80%) and ERCP (sensitivity and specificity 90%) are best. Coeliac angiography is also highly specific (174) but not very sensitive. Ultrasound or CT-guided fine needle aspiration biopsy provides a tissue diagnosis in up to 90% of cases with virtually no complications. Endoscopic ultrasound may help in tumour staging. Laparoscopy identifies 85% of the non-resectable tumours.

Differential diagnosis
Differentiate from benign adenoma of the papilla of Vater, benign cystadenoma and other pancreatic tumours.

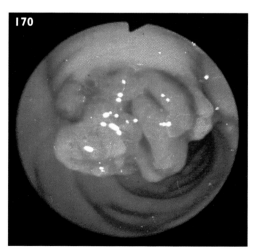

170 Carcinoma of the ampulla of Vater; this presents with obstructive jaundice and bleeding.

Cancer of the Exocrine Pancreas

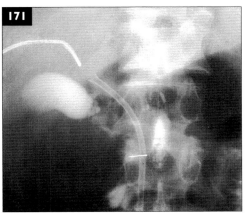

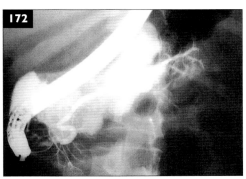

172 ERCP appearances of a patient with carcinoma of the tail of the pancreas (note truncation of the pancreatic duct).

171 Stents (inserted percutaneously along the tract outlined by the wire) are maintaining patency of the common bile duct in this patient with carcinoma of the head of the pancreas.

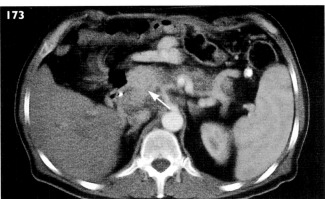

173 CT showing mass of pancreatic cancer (arrow) in the head of the pancreas.

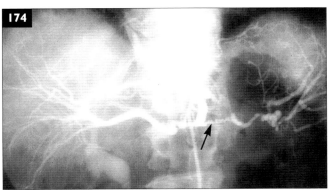

174 Coeliac angiogram in a patient with carcinoma of the pancreas. Note 'encasement' (narrowing and rigidity of the splenic artery due to carcinoma – arrow).

Cancer of the Exocrine Pancreas

Prognosis

Only 10% of the tumours are resectable. Median survival after chemotherapy is less than 20 weeks.

Management

Pancreaticoduodenectomy (Whipple's procedure) is attempted for resection, and has an operative mortality rate of 2–20%. Total pancreatectomy or other modifications may be necessary for palliation of biliary or gastrointestinal obstruction. Chemotherapy with 5-fluorouracil or mitomycin C and radiotherapy are generally ineffective. Increasingly, in elderly patients, relief of jaundice by stenting the biliary duct may be done at ERCP or by the percutaneous route under radiological control (**175, 176**). This is the mainstay of treatment. Pain relief usually requires narcotic analgesics.

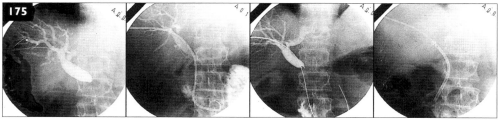

175 Pancreatic cancer causing extrahepatic obstruction. This is being relieved by the passage of a guidewire and dilatation. Subsequently, a permanent stent can be left *in situ*.

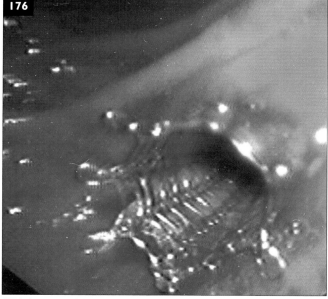

176 An expandable stent, seen from the duodenum, emerging from the bile duct where it is stenting an obstruction due to carcinoma of the pancreas.

Biliary Conditions

In the West, gallstones are the commonest cause of biliary symptomatology

Ultrasound is the mainstay of diagnosis

Obstructive jaundice merits rapid investigation, and of itself can predispose to infection in the biliary tract

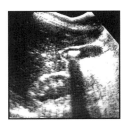 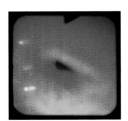 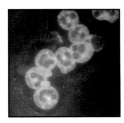 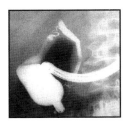

Anatomy

Intrahepatic bile ducts merge into main left and right hepatic ducts to form the common hepatic duct (**177**). This becomes the common bile duct below the origin of cystic duct, which leads into the gallbladder. Bile flow from the liver is held temporarily in the gallbladder, but passes back into the common bile duct and hence the duodenum after eating. As with other tubular organs, mucosa, submucosa and muscle layers are present.

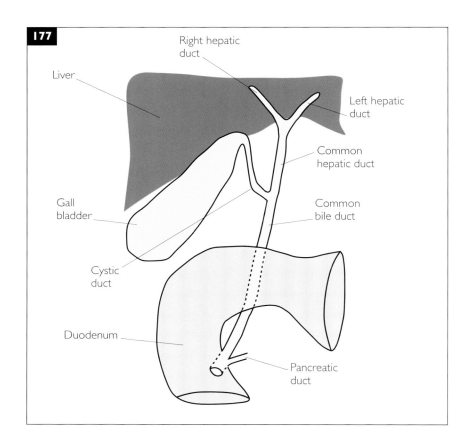

Extrahepatic Biliary Disease

The hallmark is interference with bile flow due to stasis, obstruction and/or infection. After secretion by hepatocytes into the bile canaliculi, bile is drained into enlarging ducts that eventually lead to the gallbladder and the duodenum. Specialised epithelia lining the biliary passages serve secretory, as well as absorptive functions. Common symptoms of biliary disease are jaundice, acute or recurrent upper abdominal pain, as well as fever with chills and rigors. Pathophysiologically distinct disorders include gallstone disease, benign or malignant biliary strictures, inflammatory conditions, parasitic infestations, congenital cysts, etc.

GALLSTONES
Definition
Defined as stones arising in the gallbladder. Analogous stones also occur in intrahepatic and extrahepatic biliary ducts. Manifestations range from completely asymptomatic states to biliary obstruction, infection, complications in other organs due to migration of stones, as well as increased risk for gallbladder cancer.

Epidemiology and aetiology
Gallstones are among the most common disorders, and the prevalence of gallstones has been rising. The incidence in people >40 years old is ~3% per 5-year period. Cholesterol stones are most frequently encountered (75%). Because gallstone formation is multifactorial and influenced by genetic, age-, sex- or lifestyle-specific factors, the overall prevalence significantly varies, being particularly high in Pima Indians, Caucasians in the United States and Chileans, compared with Europeans or Asians. The aphorism for gallstones of 'fat, female, fertile and forty' is not always true.

Pathophysiology
The most important elements are increased biliary cholesterol or pigment content, factors promoting nucleation of crystals, and gallbladder stasis. Diet and hepatic synthesis contribute to biliary cholesterol. Obesity, ageing, drugs and hormones may increase biliary cholesterol secretion. Free cholesterol is insoluble and bile acids and phospholipids are required for micelle formation. Deficiency of bile acid secretion or phospholipid production increase cholesterol saturation, when supersaturated cholesterol stones tend to form. Pigment stones may be 'black' or 'brown'. Black gallstones are smaller, amorphous, arise in patients with chronic haemolysis and are frequently radio-opaque. Brown stones are found in the gallbladder and bile ducts, occur in the setting of cholangitis and infection, frequently recur and are usually radiolucent.

Stone formation is aided by gallbladder stasis, as during pregnancy or total parenteral nutrition, as well as by excess mucin. 'Biliary sludge' refers to microscopic precipitates of calcium bilirubinate or cholesterol monohydrate crystals in mucin gels that are visible on ultrasound. Gallstones are increased in conditions that promote biliary sludge.

History and physical examination
Approximately two-thirds of people with gallstones are asymptomatic. Non-specific symptoms with indigestion, dyspepsia, flatulence or intolerance to fatty foods are common. More specific manifestations produce characteristic symptoms.

Biliary colic This occurs in 70–80% of symptomatic patients due to transient cystic duct spasm or obstruction. Biliary colic pain may be precipitated by a large meal, is severe and episodic in nature, located in the epigastric or right and left upper abdominal regions, may radiate to the back or shoulder, and lasts for several hours (usually <6 h).

Acute cholecystitis This is due to obstruction of the cystic duct (by gallstones in 90% of cases) Bacterial infection is usually secondary, but may produce gallbladder empyema. Acalculous acute cholecystitis occurs in 5–10% of patients in the setting of major surgery, critical illness, trauma, burns, and occasionally human immunodeficiency virus or bone marrow transplantation. The pathophysiological events in acute cholecystitis include stasis, ischaemia and necrosis. Pain lasting for >3 hours and with local tenderness, vomiting and fever is characteristic. Murphy's sign may be elicited (abrupt arrest in inspiration due to pain during abdominal palpation). In 30–40% of cases, a gallbladder and omental mass may be apparent; in 15% of cases jaundice may appear. In the elderly, only localised tenderness may be seen.

Extrahepatic Biliary Disease

Choledocholithiasis and cholangitis These conditions arise when gallstones appear in the bile ducts. Small gallstones may pass unnoticed into the duodenum, whereas large stones are entrapped in the common bile duct. Common bile duct stones are often asymptomatic (45%) or present with complications, such as biliary colic, jaundice, cholangitis and pancreatitis. Characteristic features of cholangitis are right upper quadrant pain, jaundice, chills and rigor (Charcot's triad). Impaired bile flow gives rise to 'obstructive jaundice' with itching, clay-coloured stools and biliary dilatation. In the setting of obstructive jaundice, a palpable gallbladder connotes malignancy because gallstones induce chronic cholecystitis and such a gallbladder is incapable of significant distension (Courvoisier's law). Unremitting biliary obstruction can produce secondary biliary cirrhosis within months.

Chronic cholecystitis This is due to repeated episodes of apparent or inapparent gallbladder inflammation. Right upper quadrant pain of varying severity and frequency occurs. The presentation may be coloured by associated complications, such as pancreatitis, cholangitis or choledocholithiasis.

Laboratory and special examinations
Biliary colic may be associated with no changes in blood tests. Acute cholecystitis is associated with leucocytosis, left-sided shift in neutrophils and mild increases in serum aminotransferases (~2–3-fold normal) or alkaline phosphatase (~1–2-fold normal). Biliary obstruction produces markedly elevated serum alkaline phosphatase and bilirubin levels (>70% conjugated), although obstruction due to stones is rarely complete.

Radiology Plain abdominal radiographs visualise some gallstones (13–17%). Ultrasound is highly effective (sensitivity >90%) and allows assessment of gallbladder wall thickening and sludge, intramural gas, peri-gallbladder fluid collection, biliary dilatation and gallbladder emptying (**178, 179**). Oral cholecystography has virtually been replaced by ultrasound. Radioisotope scanning with ^{99m}Tc-HIDA helps to establish gallbladder function, particularly in acute cholecystitis, as HIDA is normally taken up by the gallbladder. CT is helpful when ultrasound imaging is unsatisfactory.

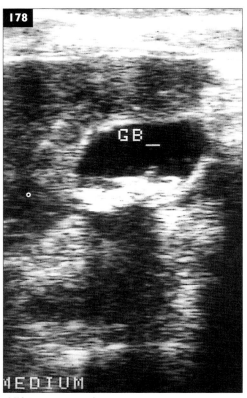

178 Ultrasound of gallbladder showing sludge and stones (casting an acoustic shadow).

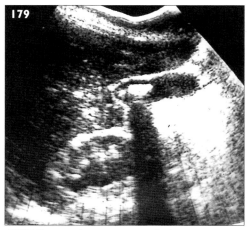

179 Ultrasound appearances of a large stone in the gallbladder with an acoustic shadow behind.

Extrahepatic Biliary Disease

The biliary tree may also be imaged by percutaneous transhepatic cholangiography (PTC) (**180**, **181**) or endoscopic retrograde cholangiography (ERC) (**182**). The former is particularly easy when bile ducts are dilated. Therapeutic interventions may be combined with either PTC or ERC, including culture or cytology of bile and insertion of draining stents.

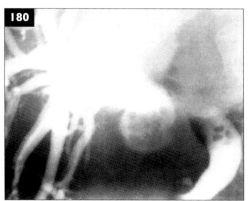

180 Percutaneous cholangiogram showing stones in the gallbladder and in the common bile duct.

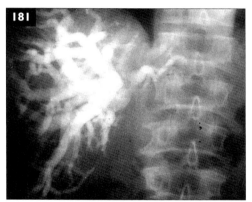

181 Carcinoma of the common hepatic duct shown on percutaneous cholangiogram with multiple dilated ducts on the right side of the liver.

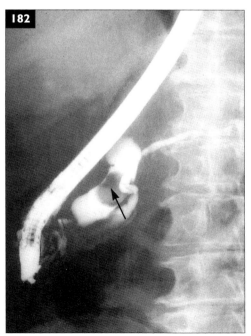

182 ERC showing a dilated common bile duct containing a large stone (arrowed).

Extrahepatic Biliary Disease

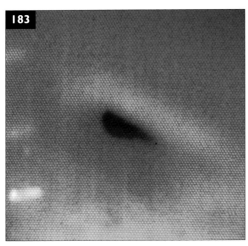

183 Appearances of the duodenum with a fistula leading into the bile duct, caused by prior passage of a stone.

Differential diagnosis

Benign gallbladder disorders may mimic cholecystitis. These include cholesterolosis (cholesterol accumulation within histiocytes in gallbladder mucosa), adenoma or adenomyomatous hyperplasia. Non-specific abdominal symptoms require distinction from oesophagitis, acid peptic disease, gastrointestinal motility disorders, irritable colon syndrome, etc. Abdominal pain may be due to renal colic, appendicitis, pancreatitis, perforated peptic ulcer, intestinal obstruction, or other conditions. Lower-lobe pneumonia, pleural or pericardial disease or coronary artery disease may also need to be considered.

Prognosis

The majority of gallstones are asymptomatic (60–80%). During a 20-year follow-up of patients, 50% remain asymptomatic, 30% develop biliary colic and 20% manifest complications. Onset of biliary colic is associated with an increased risk of complications, particularly in the diabetic, elderly or immunocompromised, such as cholangitis, pancreatitis, and gangrene or perforation of the gallbladder (10%). Acalculous disease has a poor prognosis, with a mortality rate of up to 70% in the presence of gallbladder gangrene, perforation or empyema. Other complications include pericholecystic abscess, bile peritonitis, gallstone fistula (**183**), and intestinal obstruction due to an impacted gallstone.

Management

Biliary colic is relieved with narcotic analgesics. Antibiotics active against Gram-negative microbes are necessary for treating cholangitis. Cholecystectomy is essential for acute cholecystitis, as well as for chronic cholecystitis. Laparoscopic cholecystectomy is replacing open cholecystectomy because postoperative recovery is faster. Previous abdominal surgery, diffuse peritonitis, severe obesity and pregnancy may limit laparoscopic cholecystectomy, however, and intraoperative bleeding or other complications may warrant conversion to open surgery. Gallstone dissolution by oral bile acids is limited by frequent recurrence and requirement of <1.5 cm sized, non-calcified cholesterol stones within a functioning gallbladder. Common bile duct stones may be extracted at ERCP with the aid of an endoscopic papillotomy. In selected situations, gallstones may be dissolved by administering solvents, such as methyl terbutyl ether via a T-tube placed surgically in the common bile duct or catheter placed percutaneously in the gallbladder. Extracorporeal shock wave lithotripsy has also been used to treat gallstones, although 20% of patients develop biliary colic and 10% develop pancreatitis during subsequent passage of the stone fragments.

Postcholecystectomy pain syndrome In many individuals, pain or other symptoms persist after cholecystectomy. Mild diarrhoea due to increased bile salt pool and bile salt spillage in the colon usually responds to cholestyramine. Recurrent abdominal pain (5% of cases) may be due to retained common bile duct stone, abscess, other surgical complications or unrelated cause, such as irritable colon syndrome, peptic ulcer disease, pancreatitis or biliary dyskinesia, which refers to delayed common bile duct emptying due to spasm in the sphincter of Oddi.

Choledochal Cysts

Definition
Congenital cystic malformations of the intra- or extrahepatic bile ducts. Several forms are recognised:
- Type 1, fusiform or saccular dilatation of the extrahepatic tree.
- Type 2, diverticular common bile duct cyst.
- Type 3, choledochocele.
- Type 4, diffuse dilatation of common bile duct and hepatic ducts.
- Type 5, intrahepatic ductal dilatation (Caroli's disease) (**184**).

Epidemiology and aetiology
No specific aetiology has been identified. The disorder is relatively infrequent. Most patients present in childhood, although up to 50% may present after the age of 10 years.

Pathophysiology
The cyst wall is thick, with dense connective tissue and smooth muscle. Pericystic inflammation may be noted and cholangitis is a frequent complication. Compression of the common bile duct may cause obstructive jaundice and predispose to cholangitis.

Clinical history
This ranges from asymptomatic states to jaundice, abdominal pain or fever in various combinations. Weight loss or failure to thrive is possible. Clay-coloured stools and pruritus may be prominent.

Physical examination
Look for jaundice, abdominal mass in the right upper quadrant, upper abdominal tenderness.

Laboratory and special examinations
Mild to moderate increases in serum bilirubin and alkaline phosphatase are common. Manifestations of cholangitis or obstructive jaundice may be found. Ultrasound or CT demonstrate dilated bile ducts or cystic lesions. ERC is most helpful for imaging the biliary tree and for typing.

Differential diagnosis
Distinction from biliary atresia in infants may be difficult, but critical in establishing appropriate interventions. Other conditions include liver abscess, gallstones and cancer.

Prognosis
Prognosis is usually excellent, although recurrent cholangitis may occur. Cholangiocarcinoma is more frequent in choledochal cysts.

Management
Treatment is surgical, though the specific operation depends upon the defect. Simple cystenterostomy for biliary drainage might suffice. Complete cystectomy should be undertaken for choledochal cysts.

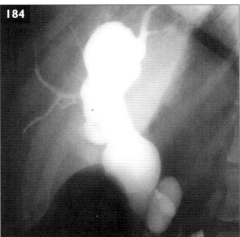

184 Gross dilatation of the extrahepatic biliary tree in Caroli's syndrome.

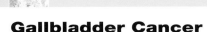

Gallbladder Cancer

Epidemiology and aetiology
Gallbladder adenocarcinoma is relatively infrequent in the West and tends to be more common in the East. There is a 3:1 greater prevalence in women. Patients tend generally to be older (>70 years) and with coexisting gallstones (80–90%). The risk factors for gallstones and gallbladder carcinoma are the same. The incidence of gallbladder carcinoma is increased with very large gallstones (>3 cm) and with gallbladder calcification producing 'porcelain gallbladder' on plain radiographs. In some cases a preneoplastic adenomatous polyp may have been identified (**185**).

Pathophysiology
Prolonged inflammation and increased epithelial cell turnover probably contribute to neoplastic transformation, although genetic changes in gallbladder carcinoma are undefined.

Clinical history
Early manifestations may be non-specific and complicated by coexisting gallstone disease. Persistent upper abdominal pain or unremitting jaundice may first indicate more serious disease. Anorexia, fatigue and weight loss may be noted.

Physical examination
Jaundice and a vaguely defined firm or hard mass in the right upper quadrant are typical.

Laboratory and special examinations
Both conjugated and unconjugated hyper-bilirubinaemia are present due to a combination of biliary obstruction and hepatic dysfunction. Other manifestations may include low serum albumin, prolonged prothrombin time and elevated serum alkaline phosphatase. Ultrasound or CT imaging demonstrate gallbladder lesions (**186, 187**), commonly accompanied by liver metastases. The diagnosis may also be indicated by ERC or PTC. Endoscopic ultrasound and angiography may be helpful for staging. Fine needle aspiration biopsy could establish tissue diagnosis.

Differential diagnosis
Differentiate from other causes of obstructive or mixed cholestatic/hepatocellular-type jaundice.

Prognosis
Gallbladder carcinoma can be resected in only <20% of cases. Disease commonly extends to bile ducts, liver, portal lymph nodes, as well as to distant organs. In the presence of jaundice, gallbladder carcinoma is unresectable in >85% of patients.

Management
Chemotherapy or radiotherapy are ineffective. Care is usually aimed at symptomatic palliation, including relief of biliary obstruction by internal stents.

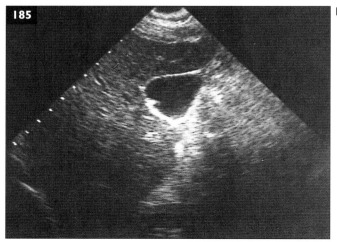

185 A small gallbladder polyp (non-mobile) is seen protruding from the wall. Although usually benign, they have the propensity to develop into malignant tumours.

Gallbladder Cancer

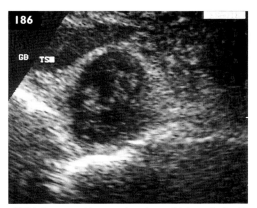

186 Ultrasound image showing a thick-walled gall gladder containing tumour.

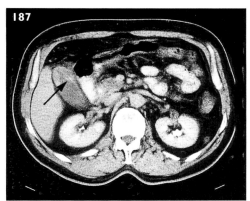

187 CT image (same patient) showing thick-walled gall bladder (arrowed) infiltrated by cancer.

Cholangiohepatitis

Definition
Defined as recurrent episodes of cholangitis due to intrahepatic bile duct stones, often in conjunction with parasitic infestation.

Epidemiology and aetiology
The condition is most frequently encountered in South-east Asia (50–80%) and only rarely in Western countries (0.6–2.4%). Patients tend to be younger than those with gallbladder stones, from poor socioeconomic situations, and frequently suffer from malnutrition. Associated parasitic infestations include *Clonorchis sinensis* (25%) and Ascariasis (13–20%). Gallbladder stones may coexist in 33% of the patients.

Pathophysiology
Parasites in intrahepatic bile ducts interfere with biliary drainage, induce recurrent episodes of cholangitis, and excite the host immune response with hepatic fibrosis, bile duct proliferation, dilatation, as well as suppuration. Black pigment stones containing calcium bilirubinate are frequent.

Clinical history
Recurrent pain, fever and jaundice occurring at intervals of weeks, months or years are typical.

Physical examination
Look for jaundice, hepatomegaly (19% of cases) and a palpable gallbladder (9%).

Laboratory and special examinations
Plain radiograph of the abdomen is unhelpful. CT tends to be more helpful than ultrasound in demonstrating calcific lesions or hepatic abnormalities. ERCP or PTC are most helpful in diagnosis. Biliary strictures are frequent (35%) and most commonly involve the left hepatic duct (90%).

Differential diagnosis
Differentiate from other causes of cholangitis.

Prognosis
Prognosis depends upon the duration of symptoms, and the severity of biliary strictures and liver disease. Mortality rates within 1 month of surgical therapy approach 4–10% and increase progressively with multiple surgical interventions. Acalculous cholecystitis (40% of cases) is often severe and may prove fatal.

Management
The mainstays are surgery and endoscopic intervention, the goals being to remove ductal stones, drain obstructed segments of the bile ducts, and dilate strictures. Eradication of parasites may not arrest or reverse disease.

Primary Sclerosing Cholangitis (PSC)

Definition
Insidious and progressive inflammatory disorder with immunological abnormalities resulting in fibrosis and segmental obliteration of large bile ducts.

Epidemiology and aetiology
The cause is unknown. A strong association exists with inflammatory bowel disease (IBD) and PSC occurs in approximately 3–5% of all patients with IBD. Up to 50% of PSC patients may manifest with IBD, and if fully investigated to detect subclinical disease, 80–90% of patients may be shown to have IBD, and the proportion will rise with time. The IBD is much more commonly ulcerative colitis than Crohn's disease. However, PSC does not remit after colectomy and there is no correlation between disease activity of IBD and PSC. The prevalence of human leucocyte antigens (HLA) B8 and DR3 is increased in PSC.

Pathophysiology
A variety of immunological abnormalities have been noted, but the precise significance of these observations remains unclear. Autoantibodies have been identified directed against shared antigens displayed on colon and biliary epithelial cells. Liver biopsy demonstrates periportal accumulation of small and large lymphocytes, periductular inflammation and destruction, as well as 'onion-skin' liver fibrosis (**188**).

Clinical history
This ranges from insidious onset of chronic cholestasis to recurrent episodes of cholangitis (15–20% of cases). Pruritus, weight loss, fatigue and malaise may be noted. An isolated increase in serum alkaline phosphatase levels may antedate symptoms by months to years.

Physical examination
The liver may be normal in size to mildly enlarged. Splenomegaly and ascites may develop in late stages due to portal hypertension.

Laboratory and special examinations
Biochemical parameters are indicative of cholangitis or cholestasis. The diagnosis is best established by demonstration of characteristic morphological changes in bile ducts by ERCP (**189**) or PTC. Liver biopsy may also be diagnostic. A characteristic autoantibody (anti-neutrophil cytoplasmic antibody, ANCA) can generally be found in the circulation (**190**).

Differential diagnosis
Differentiate from other cholestatic disorders, including primary biliary cirrhosis. Benign biliary strictures may arise from trauma, infection, ischaemia, and hepatic arterial chemotherapy. Recurrent infection in the setting of benign strictures can lead to secondary sclerosing cholangitis. Infectious cholangiopathy in the setting of acquired immunodeficiency syndrome (cryptosporidia or microsporidia) may need to be distinguished.

Prognosis
The most important prognostic indicators are age, serum bilirubin, liver histology and the presence or absence of splenomegaly. Untreated, patients with PSC demonstrate progressive deterioration over a prolonged period of 10–20 years, ultimately with hepatic failure. Cholangiocarcinoma is a frequent complication (20–30%).

Management
No specific therapies are available. The mainstays are antibiotics for symptomatic bacterial cholangitis, and endoscopic dilatation of accessible strictures. Anti-inflammatory therapies, including corticosteroids, azathioprine, methotrexate and others, have been used. Ursodeoxycholic acid may improve pruritus, as well as biochemical parameters. Prolonged cholestasis may be accompanied by deficiencies of fat-soluble vitamins and appropriate supplements, particularly to prevent bone disease, are necessary. Distinctions between stricturing lesions and cholangio-carcinoma may be particularly difficult and require brush cytology, as well as biopsy. Orthotopic liver transplantation in advanced disease provides excellent outcomes.

Primary Sclerosing Cholangitis (PSC)

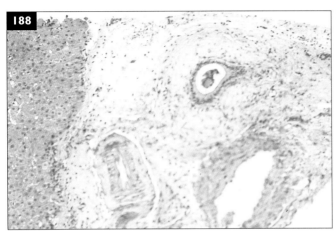

188 Liver biopsy appearances in sclerosing cholangitis showing 'onion skin' fibrosis around the bile ducts.

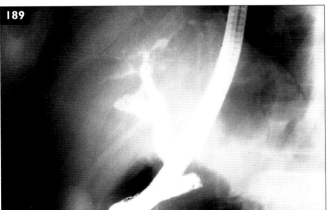

189 ERCP examination of the liver showing truncated irregular intrahepatic bile ducts in primary sclerosing cholangitis.

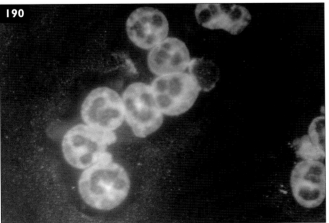

190 ANCA-anti-neutrophil cytoplasmic antibody – an autoantibody in the serum of most patients with sclerosing cholangitis, detected by immunofluorescence on normal neutrophils.

Cholangiocarcinoma

Definition
Adenocarcinoma originating in the biliary epithelium.

Epidemiology and aetiology
Overall, males are more frequently affected. Cholangiocarcinoma is more prevalent in the Far East in the setting of cholangiohepatitis, and also occurs in primary sclerosing cholangitis and choledochal cysts.

Pathophysiology
Polypoid, sclerosing or infiltrating tumours. Poorly defined thickening of bile duct wall leads to luminal narrowing, often resembling fibrous strictures or sclerosing cholangitis. Tumours are slow-growing, with a tendency for infiltration of duct wall, and spread to lymph nodes. The tumours may be located within or outside the liver, and may locate at the junction of the right and left hepatic bile ducts (Klatskin tumour).

Clinical history
Vague upper abdominal pain, asymptomatic increase in serum alkaline phosphatase without jaundice, progressive obstructive jaundice or cholangitis.

Physical examination
Mild hepatomegaly in the presence of obstructive jaundice. Ill-defined upper abdominal mass in advanced stages.

Laboratory and special examinations
Biochemical findings are non-specific and consistent with partial or total biliary obstruction. Ultrasound, CT or percutaneous cholangiography (191) may demonstrate dilated intrahepatic bile ducts along with focal narrowing in the biliary tree. A heterogeneous hepatic mass may be apparent. ERCP permits precise localisation of the biliary abnormality (192), as well as cytology of the aspirated bile or brushings. Needle aspiration biopsy may be helpful.

Differential diagnosis
Differentiate from benign biliary strictures, primary sclerosing cholangitis, pancreatic carcinoma, lesions of the ampulla of Vater, hepatocellular carcinoma, lymph node metastases in the porta hepatis, and other cholestatic disorders.

Prognosis
At laparotomy, only one-third of the tumours are resectable. The 5-year survival rate after attempted resection is only ~20%. Most patients die of hepatic invasion and liver failure.

Management
Resection is usually not possible. Chemotherapy or external radiotherapy are generally ineffective, although brachytherapy (intraductal radiation by implanted sources) shows some promise. Orthotopic liver transplantation for intrahepatic cholangiocarcinoma has been very disappointing due to early recurrence.

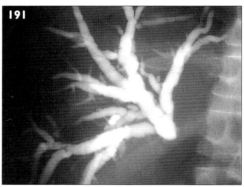

191 Percutaneous cholangiogram showing dilated ducts. There is an abrupt cut-off at the top of the common hepatic duct, due to the presence of a cholangiocarcinoma.

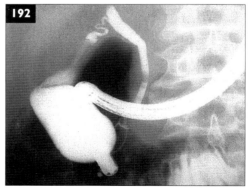

192 ERCP shows filling of common bile duct, gall bladder, and common hepatic duct. but above this there is a blind upper end of the common hepatic duct due to a cholangiocarcinoma.

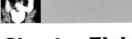

Chapter Eight

Colonic Disease

Colonic cancer is common. As there are generally many years of benign adenomatous growth before malignancy occurs, it is also preventable

Ulcerative colitis can present as a medical emergency and urgent treatment may avoid the need for colectomy

Colonoscopy and biopsy are the most effective diagnostic manoeuvres

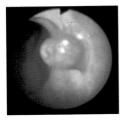 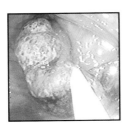 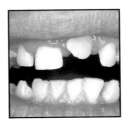 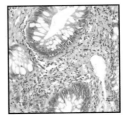

Anatomy

The colon is approximately 1.5 metres long, commencing in the right iliac fossa at the ileocaecal valve, and consists of the caecum, ascending colon, transverse colon, descending colon, sigmoid, and rectum.

The transverse colon and sigmoid colon are particularly mobile on a free mesentery, while the caecum, ascending colon, and descending colon are relatively fixed without a free mesentery. The lower 12 cm of the rectum lie below the peritoneal reflection.

INVESTIGATIONS

The two major investigations of the colon are:
- Barium enema: this is best performed after a few days on a low-residue diet, and emptying the colon by either laxatives of colonic lavage. Barium is run in, evacuated, and air insufflated, to give single and air-contrast barium enemas (**193**). The procedure should not be performed if there is active inflammatory bowel disease of more than mild severity.
- Endoscopy: rigid sigmoidoscopy visualises the lowest 12–28 cm of the bowel, and biopsies can be taken. No preparation is needed. The technique is useful for assessing the presence/activity of ulcerative colitis.

Flexible sigmoidoscopy visualises the left side of the colon; a simple enema to empty the colon is generally needed. It is useful for investigating some forms of rectal bleeding, and convenient for cancer screening as the majority of tumours/polyps are left-sided, and the procedure is quicker and more convenient than full colonoscopy. However, this is a compromise!

Colonoscopy (**194**) visualises the whole of the colon (unless the bowel is very tortuous) and often the terminal ileum can be entered. A full preparation to empty the bowel is required.

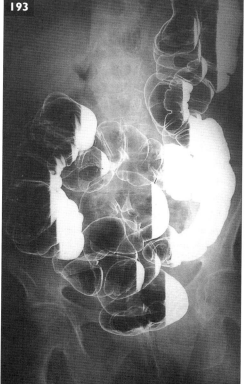

193 Normal barium enema (taken in left lateral decubitus position) showing distinction between air contrast and barium contrast.

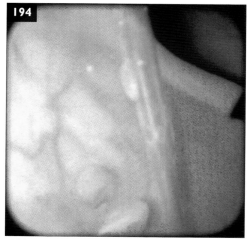

194 Normal appearances of caecum (including tomato debris) This demonstrates the normal vascular pattern.

Anatomy

Both flexible sigmoidoscopy and colonoscopy allow multiple biopsies to be taken. Special techniques (magnifying colonoscopes, spraying the mucosa with dye) may help to identify very small areas of abnormality.

The correct procedure to use varies and the procedures are complementary.

For pain, a barium enema may be the better procedure: for bleeding, colonoscopy is better as it offers the opportunity of therapy, i.e. snaring of colonic polyps.

Other investigations

- Plain X-ray (**195 & 196**). Displays the presence/absence of colonic dilatation, obstruction, and volvulus, and is often helpful in delineating the extent of inflammatory colitis.
- Labelled leucocyte scanning – identifies areas of inflammation (e.g. ulcerative colitis, Crohn's disease, pseudomembranous colitis).
- Anorectal manometry – for investigation of incontinence or severe constipation.

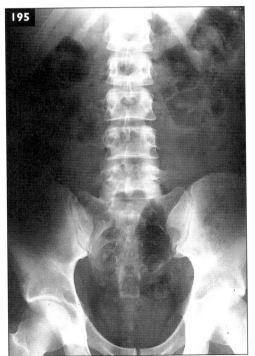

195 Plain X-ray – sparse air-filling of the colon shows normal, non-dilated large bowel.

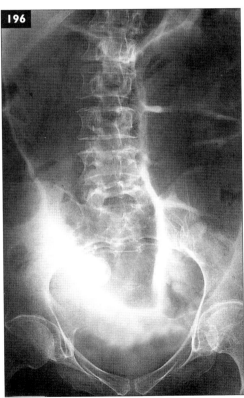

196 Sigmoid volvulus showing grossly dilated colon extending from left of pelvis and giving the typical 'coffee bean' appearance.

Colonic Polyps

Definition
Polyps are abnormal structures that arise from the gastrointestinal mucosa and protrude into the lumen (**197, 198**). The colonic polyps may be single or multiple, sessile or pedunculated and sporadic or hereditary in origin.

Epidemiology and aetiology
The origin of colonic polyps is multifactorial. Several histological types are recognised:
- Hyperplastic polyps: these are characterised by metaplastic change, but have no neoplastic potential. These polyps are small, asymptomatic, usually found at endoscopy, mostly located in the rectum and distal sigmoid colon, and are frequent (20% of all polyps).
- Inflammatory polyps: these are also non-neoplastic, arise in the setting of chronic mucosal inflammation, e.g. ulcerative colitis, and are restricted to areas of the inflamed bowel.
- Juvenile polyps: these are hamartomas of the lamina propria, may be single or multiple, are mostly situated in the rectum and may present with haemorrhage or autoamputation.
- Adenomatous polyps: these are neoplastic and thus of the greatest concern.

The incidence of adenomatous polyps increases with age and parallels the risk for colon carcinoma. In the United States, colon polyps are present in 40–50% of people aged over 60 years. In contrast, colon polyps are infrequent in populations at low risk for colon carcinoma, e.g. in South African Blacks (<0.5%) or Japanese people (10%). The risk of colon carcinoma in patients with polyps is related to the size and not to the number of polyps. Adenomatous polyps may be tubular (60%; small, spherical, stalk present, lobulated surface), villous (10%; large, sessile, velvety surface with fronds), or tubulovillous (30%; hybrid features). All adenomatous polyps display dysplastic changes with nuclear abnormalities, as well as a glandular architecture. Several genetic disorders are recognised with specific chromosomal abnormalities leading to colonic polyps.

Pathophysiology
The colonic epithelium is normally replenished every 3–8 days with migration of proliferating cells from the bottom of the mucosal crypts toward the surface. In adenomas, cellular DNA synthesis is amplified, immature epithelial cells are found in the crypts closer to the mucosal surface, and proliferating cells accumulate on the luminal surface, producing new adenomatous tissues. The relationship between adenomatous polyps and colon carcinoma was deduced from their similar epidemiological features and anatomical distributions, presence of adenomatous tissue in small cancers, adenoma–carcinoma transition in familial polyposis syndromes, decrease in the risk of colon cancer after removal of polyps and a lag period of several years between the onset of polyps and progression to malignancy.

Clinical history
Most polyps are asymptomatic. Occult blood in the stool is frequent. Rectal bleeding is occasionally reported.

Physical examination
Polyps may sometimes be palpable on rectal examination. Screening sigmoidoscopy may demonstrate silent polyps.

Laboratory and special examinations
A blood count and iron studies may unmask an iron-deficiency anaemia. Polyps may be demonstrated by double-contrast barium enema (sensitivity 80–90%). Flexible sigmoidoscopy and colonoscopy are more sensitive (up to 98%) and provide the added advantage of biopsy or removal.

Differential diagnosis
Distinction to be made between various types of polyps and colon cancer.

Prognosis
Colon carcinoma occurs in 1–3%, 10% and 40% of polyps with sizes of <1 cm, 1–2 cm and >2 cm, respectively. Villous adenomas are most frequently malignant (40%) followed by tubulovillous (23%) and tubular (<5%) adenomas. Adenomatous polyps have a tendency to recur and prolonged surveillance is required. The prognosis is worse in the presence of poorly differentiated polyps, penetration of muscularis mucosae, vascular or lymphatic invasion and cancer in the resection margin.

Management
The majority of colonic polyps are removed or destroyed by endoscopic procedures, such as a 'hot biopsy' or snare diathermy using electrocautery (**199, 200**). Surgery is only rarely necessary. As new adenomatous polyps tend to develop, colonoscopy is performed 1 year after polyp removal and when no further polyps are found, at 3- to 5-year intervals.

Colonic Polyps

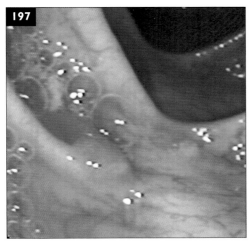

197 Small sessible polyp.

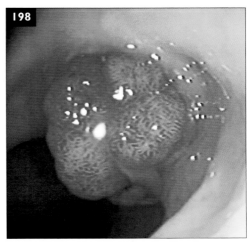

198 Polyp in sigmoid colon.

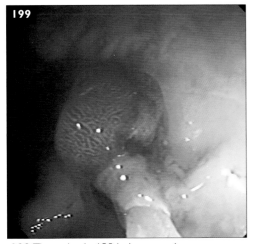

199 The polyp in 198 being snared.

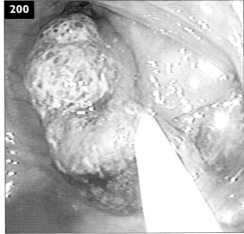

200 Large colonic polyp being snared.

Colon Carcinoma

Definition
Adenocarcinoma originating in the large intestine and rectum.

Epidemiology and aetiology
Colon carcinoma is frequent in North America, north-western Europe and New Zealand, but less common in South America, south-east Asia, equatorial Africa and India. In the UK there are 18 000 new cases per year and 13 000 deaths. The incidence increases in people after migration from low- to high-incidence areas. The genetic mechanisms involve chromosomes 17 and 18 with the 'Deleted in Colon Carcinoma (DCC)' gene and the 'Nucleotide mismatch repair' gene, as well as protooncogene abnormalities, such as in c-*myc*, c-*Ki-ras* and *p53* genes. The nucleotide mismatch repair gene abnormalities are transmitted as autosomal dominant with a high penetrance (hereditary non-polyposis, carcinoma of the colon, HNPCC). Low intake of dietary fibre, calcium or vitamin D, excess consumption of saturated animal fats and obesity increase risk, whereas high consumption of anticarcinogens in fruits and vegetables may decrease risk. Intake of aspirin and non-steroidal anti-inflammatory agents appears to protect against colon cancer. Other risk factors are age over 50 years, long-standing ulcerative colitis or Crohn's disease, past history of colon adenoma or cancer, breast and female genital tract cancer (Lynch II syndrome), and family history of polyposis syndromes or colorectal carcinoma.

Pathophysiology
Colonic adenocarcinoma most commonly follows the polyp–adenoma– carcinoma sequence involving uncontrolled cell proliferation in epithelial crypts. There is varying glandular differentiation and mucin production. Right-sided colonic tumours are more frequently polypoid and left-sided tumours annular or constricting. The last 60 cm of the colon harbour 50% of the tumours. The descending colon, sigmoid colon and rectum contain most tumours (75%), followed by caecum and ascending colon (15%) and transverse colon (10%). Tumours spread by direct extension into pericolonic fat, mesentery, surrounding organs and the peritoneal cavity, by lymphatics to the lymph nodes, and via the portal vein to the liver.

Clinical history
Rectal bleeding, change in bowel habit, colonic obstruction, and iron-deficiency anaemia each are common presentations. Right-sided tumours are more likely to present with anaemia, left-sided with frank bleeding or obstruction. Pedigree analysis is helpful when appropriate.

Physical examination
A rectal mass may be digitally palpated. Signs of liver disease, localised perforation, peritonitis and abdominal masses may be noted. Manifestations may be of distant metastases.

Laboratory and special examinations
Biochemical and haematological tests are non-diagnostic. Serum carcinoembryonic antigen (CEA) is of no value in screening. Flexible sigmoidoscopy (**201**) plus double-contrast barium enema (**202** and **203**) may often be adequate. A colonoscopy is necessary for tissue diagnosis of lesions proximal to the descending colon (**204**). Imaging modalities, including chest radiograph, CT and endoscopic ultrasound, may be helpful for tumour staging.

Differential diagnosis
Differentiate from carcinoma of the anal canal: lymphoma, leiomyosarcoma, malignant carcinoid, Kaposi's sarcoma; differentiate also from invasion of cancers from adjacent organs (prostate, ovary, uterus or stomach). Benign lesions that may mimic colonic cancer include benign polyps, lipoma of the ileocaecal valve and others.

Prognosis
The 10-year survival rate after resection approaches ~40%. Survival is dependent upon tumour staging (Dukes' classification and TNM classification are both used).

Dukes' class A (confined to mucosa), B (extending through all areas of bowel wall) and C (regional lymph nodes) are associated with 5-year survival rate of 80–90%, 70–80% and 30–55%, respectively.

The TNM stages O (*in situ* cancer), I (limited to the mucosa, submucosa or external muscle), II (penetration of all adjacent bowel layers), III (spread to regional lymph nodes, nearby tissues or organs), and IV (distant sites, e.g. liver, lungs) are associated with generally similar outcomes.

Early detection and removal of adenomatous colonic polyps is the most effective means of improving prognosis. A total colonoscopy should be performed before surgery for detecting synchronous lesions elsewhere. Surveillance to detect recurrent polyps after surgery for colon cancer uses stool occult blood testing and

Colon Carcinoma

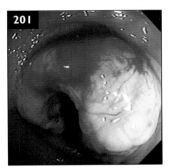

201 Carcinoma in the rectosigmoid.

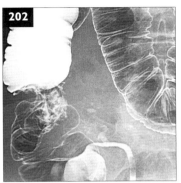

202 Barium X-ray showing an 'apple core' lesion in the ascending colon.

203 Barium X-ray of the rectum showing a polypoid tumour low in the rectal canal.

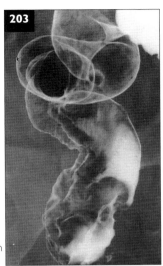

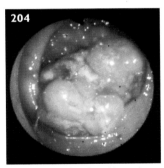

204 A caecal polypoid carcinoma.

colonoscopy within 2–3 months, 1 year later and every 3 years subsequently. The roles of periodic chest radiograph, abdominal CT or serum CEA levels to detect asymptomatic metastatic disease are unclear.

Management

A multidisciplinary approach is essential. The affected segment, omentum and lymph nodes are resected. A hemicolectomy is necessary for right- or left-sided lesions. Lesions in the sigmoid colon and rectum are resected with wide margins. Solitary hepatic metastases may be amenable to surgical resection. In advanced cancer, only palliative therapy may be practical, such as a decompressive colostomy or laser photoablation to relieve obstruction. Chemotherapeutic regimens most often employ cyclical 5-fluorouracil and levamisole and appear to improve outcome. Combination radiotherapy with up to 50 Gy may be given. Adjuvant chemotherapy (5-fluorouracil plus levamisole or leucovorin) is given for lymph node involvement and improves survival if given in less advanced disease. Floxuridine has been infused into the hepatic artery for metastatic disease. Rectal carcinoma and anal carcinoma are treated by a combination of radiotherapy and chemotherapy.

Prevention

To prevent colon cancer, a number of different strategies can be adopted. Routine screening of the middle-aged population can define the presence of polyps, or early cancers, after faecal occult blood screening or routine endoscopy (flexible sigmoidoscopy, rigid sigmoidoscopy and full colonoscopy have all been advocated). Such approaches are expensive.

High-risk groups (previous polyps, family history of cancer at an early age or in more than one relative) can be screened with a higher yield of malignant or pre-malignant disease.

Some dietary habits (high calcium intake, high fibre, less red meat) may be preventative and are under assessment, as is continuous low-dose acetylsalicylic acid orally.

Polyposis Syndromes – Mainly Inherited

FAMILIAL ADENOMATOUS POLYPOSIS
This disorder is transmitted in an autosomal dominant fashion with high penetrance. The adenomatous polyposis coli (APC) gene is located on chromosome 5. Colon polyps begin to appear in early teens and gastrointestinal symptoms in the third or fourth decades of life. The colon is studded with hundreds or thousands of polyps (**205–207**), and colon carcinoma develops by the age of 40 in virtually all patients. Upper gastrointestinal polyps are common (stomach (**208**), mostly hyperplastic polyps; duodenum, 80% adenomatous polyps with periampullary carcinoma in 10%). Eye lesions (Conjunctival Hypertrophy of Retinal Pigment Epithelium, CHRPE, **209**) are found in 80% of patients. A subtype of familial polyposis, the Gardner syndrome, is characterised by benign extraintestinal growths, osteomas (mandibular), soft tissue tumours (lipomas, sebaceous cysts, fibrosarcomas), supernumerary teeth (**210**), desmoid tumours (**211**) and mesenteric fibromatosis. Colectomy is indicated when polyps appear in individuals with familial adenomatous polyposis. Until recently, flexible sigmoidoscopy on an annual basis has been deemed necessary in

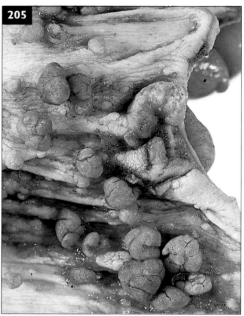

205 Resection specimen of the colon showing multiple polyps and familial polyposis.

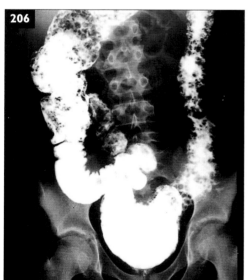

206 Familial polyposis on single contrast barium enema. Note the numerous rounded polypoid filling defects, particularly in the ascending colon.

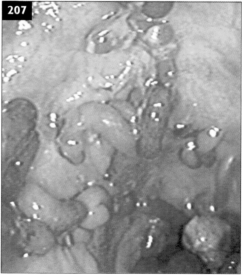

207 Multiple polyps should always be biopsied to differentiate neoplastic adenomatous polyps from regenerative polyps.

Polyposis Syndromes – Mainly Inherited

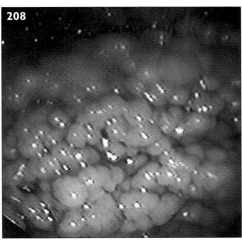

208 Endoscopic appearances of gastric mucosa in familial polyposis showing multiple polyps.

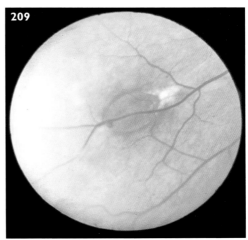

209 Fundoscopy showing congenital hypertrophy of the retinal pigment epithelium (CHRPE).

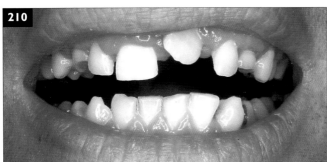

210 Abnormal dentition in familial polyposis coli.

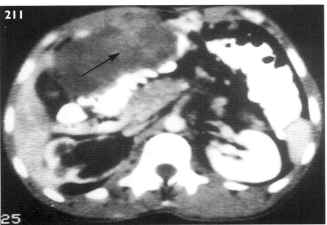

211 Some patients with familial polyposis coli have desmoid tumours. This intra-abdominal desmoid (arrow) is compressing the small intestine.

Polyposis Syndromes – Mainly Inherited

all first-degree relatives between the ages of 12 and 40 years and every 3 years subsequently. Genetic analysis for mutations may in future allow relatives to be 'cleared' from risk. Endoscopic surveillance for gastric and duodenal polyps is recommended every 2–3 years when colonic polyps develop. Additional interventions depending upon complications may be required by patients with Gardner syndrome.

TURCOT'S SYNDROME
An autosomal recessive or dominant disorder with abnormalities in the APC gene plus the nucleotide mismatch repair gene. The disorder is rare. Characteristic features are a lower number of colon polyps (20–300) and central nervous tumours, such as medulloblastoma, glioblastoma and ependymoma.

PEUTZ–JEGHER'S SYNDROME
This is transmitted as autosomal dominant with variable penetrance. Hamartomatous polyps may extend from the stomach to the rectum. Melanotic spots are found in lips, buccal mucosa and skin. Polyps are relatively sparse and exhibit a branching glandular pattern with smooth muscle proliferation. Presentations are of gastro-intestinal bleeding, colicky abdominal pain and intussusception. Rare associations include small-intestinal malignancy, ovarian stromal tumours, and gallbladder, ureteric or nasal polyps.

JUVENILE POLYPOSIS
This is usually transmitted as an autosomal dominant disorder but occasionally in a sporadic manner. Polyps number 25–40 and may be either restricted to the colon or involve the entire gastrointestinal tract. Rectal bleeding, iron deficiency anaemia, abdominal pain or intussusception may be presenting features in early childhood or adolescence. Congenital malformations may be noted, including pulmonary arteriovenous malformations. Approximately 10% develop gastrointestinal cancer. Subtotal colectomy is often necessary.

CRONKHITE–CANADA SYNDROME
A non-familial disorder affecting adults. Polyps are commonly distributed in the stomach and colon. Other features are alopecia, fingernail dystrophy and cutaneous hyperpigmentation. Watery diarrhoea, anorexia, abdominal pain, cachexia and protein-losing enteropathy are manifestations, with gastrointestinal cancers in 14%.

COWDEN'S SYNDROME
An autosomal dominant disorder with multiple hamartomas, facial tricholemmomas, oral papillomas (**212**), keratoses of the hands and feet, non-dysplastic colonic polyps without increase in colon cancer but with malignancy in other organs, e.g. thyroid and breast.

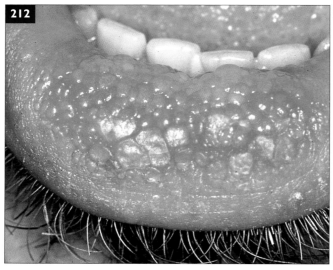

212 A patient with Cowden's syndrome.

Ulcerative Colitis

Definition
This is a chronic inflammatory condition of unknown aetiology affecting a portion or all of the colon (213, 214). Ulcerative colitis may on occasion be indistinguishable from Crohn's colitis.

Epidemiology and aetiology
Although genetic and immunologic mechanisms play important roles, the precise aetiology remains unknown. The disease afflicts all age groups with a bimodal distribution, peaking between the second and third decades (the majority) or sixth and eighth decades. Ulcerative colitis is most common in Northern Europe and America, as well as in European emigrants elsewhere. Ashkenazi Jews originating in Europe, compared with Sephardim, are more often affected. Ulcerative colitis is rare in central or south America, Africa, the Middle East and Asia. However, no ethnic group is immune and the incidence of ulcerative colitis increases in black, Hispanic or Asian immigrants domiciled in high incidence areas. Inflammatory bowel disease may show clustering in families. Offspring of two parents with the disease have a significant (40–50%) chance of acquiring inflammatory bowel disease. No specific genetic mode of transmission, however, has been identified. Cigarette smoking may protect against ulcerative colitis and indeed colitis may develop for the first time upon cessation of smoking. Environmental factors, including colonic bacteria, are most likely involved in inflammatory bowel disease.

Pathophysiology
In the mucosa in ulcerative colitis there are multiple pro-inflammatory processes, such as T-cell proliferation, antibody production, as well as expression of inflammatory mediators, such as leukotrienes, platelet-activating factor, histamine, kinins, chemotactic substances and neuropeptides. The end result is mucosal inflammation, exudation

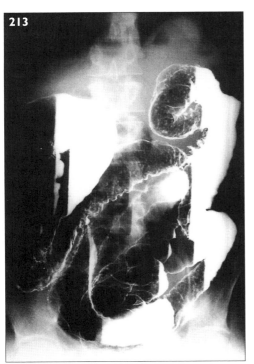

213 Barium enema showing diffuse ulcerative colitis with multiple ulcers and a shaggy irregular mucosa.

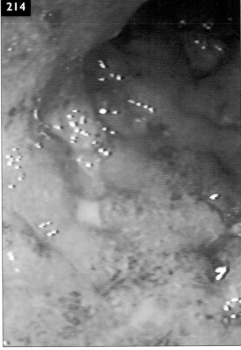

214 Endoscopic appearance of acute ulcerative colitis.

Ulcerative Colitis

of an inflammatory infiltrate containing neutrophils, epithelial necrosis and ulceration (215–219). The inflammatory infiltrate is most pronounced in the lamina propria and epithelium, without being transmural. Accumulation of the inflammatory exudate between adjacent crypts generates 'crypt abscesses' and goblet cells are depleted of mucus. Repeated injury and repair ultimately lead to fibrosis and thinning of the colonic wall, loss of haustrations (lead pipe appearance) and development occasionally of strictures. Areas of hyperplastic mucosa in the setting of ongoing inflammation appear as 'pseudopolyps' at endoscopy (220). Mucosal cells may demonstrate nuclear atypia (dysplastic change) (221) with an increased risk for colon carcinoma.

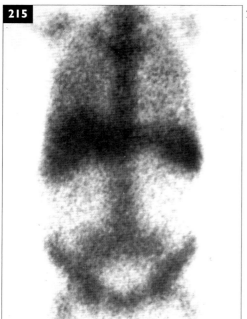

215 A negative white cell scan showing the normal distribution of labelled leucocytes to liver, spleen and bone marrow.

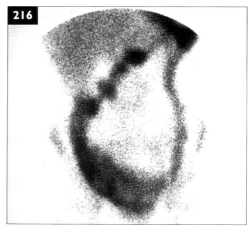

216 White cell scan showing diffuse inflammation throughout the transverse, descending colon and the rectum in active pancolitis.

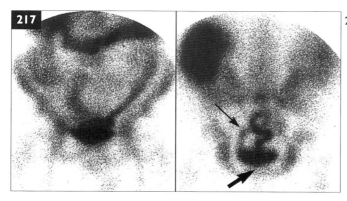

217 White cell scan showing accumulation of neutrophils throughout the ascending colon, transverse colon, descending colon and the pelvis of a patient with colitis (left panel). Because the isotope is also excreted into the bladder, a pelvic outlet view (right panel) shows the bladder anteriorly (thick arrow) and the rectum behind that (fine arrow).

Ulcerative Colitis

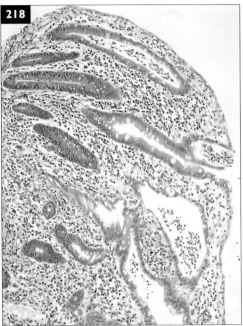

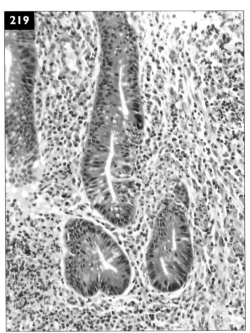

218 Biopsy specimen of acute ulcerative colitis showing diffuse inflammatory infiltrate, loss of surface epithelium, loss of mucin and crypt abscesses (neutrophils in the gland spaces).

219 Histological section of active ulcerative colitis Note the distorted gland architecture and branching glands, indicating that regeneration has taken place.

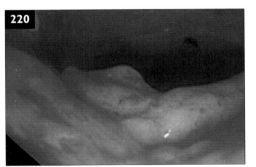

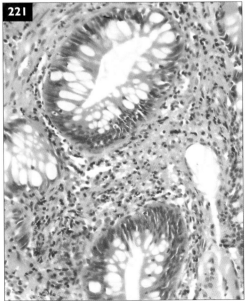

220 Endoscopic appearance of pseudopolyp (regenerative epithelium).

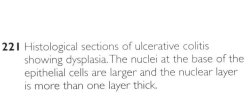

221 Histological sections of ulcerative colitis showing dysplasia. The nuclei at the base of the epithelial cells are larger and the nuclear layer is more than one layer thick.

Ulcerative Colitis

Left-sided colitis involving the rectum and sigmoid colon is most frequent (25–50%); the rectum alone may be involved (25%), or inflammation may extend proximal to the splenic flexure and produce pancolitis (25–30%) (**222, 223**). Occasionally, proctitis may accompany patches of colitis in the caecum or right colon. The inflamed segments of the colon are diffusely involved in contrast to discontinuous involvement and skip areas in Crohn's colitis. The ileum is not affected in ulcerative colitis, although inflammatory exudate may flow into the ileum producing so-called 'backwash ileitis'.

Clinical history
The onset of an attack is usually insidious, depending upon disease extent and severity. Proctitis manifests with tenesmus and semi-solid stool containing blood, mucus and pus. Diarrhoea, abdominal pain, cramping or distension and localised tenderness are additional features of more extensive disease. Systemic symptoms may occur, such as fever, malaise, nausea, vomiting, night sweats and arthralgias. Coexisting constipation or irritable colon syndrome may mask manifestations of ulcerative colitis. Severe colitis is characterised by increased bowel frequency, blood in stool, fever, tachycardia, anaemia, rising ESR, marked abdominal tenderness, decreased bowel sounds and colonic dilatation. Clinical features of severe disease (*Table 3*) indicate that a patient should be admitted to hospital for treatment, including notably the use of intravenous steroids.

Physical examination
There may be evidence of weight loss, eye abnormalities such as uveitis, skin rashes, pyoderma gangrenosum, arthritis, finger clubbing, localised or diffuse abdominal tenderness with or without abdominal distension.

Laboratory and special examinations
With increasing severity and length of relapses, there may be peripheral leucocytosis, anaemia of chronic disease or of iron deficiency, thrombocythaemia, fluid and electrolyte imbalances, (particularly hypokalaemia), hypoalbuminaemia secondary to protein-losing enteropathy, evidence of systemic inflammation (raised ESR, acute phase response proteins), elevated serum alkaline phosphatase, amino-transferases or GGT in case of coexisting hepatitis or cholangitis. Plain radiograph of abdomen may demonstrate toxic megacolon (transverse colon >6 cm) (**224**) or colonic

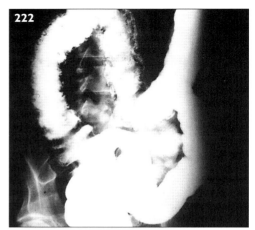

222 Single contrast barium enema showing pancolitis. Note the undermining 'collar-stud' ulcers in the transverse colon.

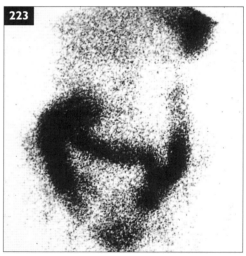

223 Pancolitis with leucocytes attracted to the whole of the colon.

Table 3. Clinical characteristics of severe colitis

Diarrhoea	Six times daily
Macroscopic blood	+++
Temperature	>38°C
Pulse	>100/min
ESR	>30 mm/h
Hb	<11 G/dl

Ulcerative Colitis

perforation (free air under the diaphragm). A barium enema may demonstrate mucosal ulceration or irregularity and colonic shortening with loss of haustral pattern in chronic disease (**213, 222, 225, 226**). Barium enema is ill-advised in acute colitis as it may precipitate toxic megacolon (see below). Sigmoidoscopy and rectal biopsy are extremely helpful for demonstrating characteristic endoscopic

and histological features. The mucosa is diffusely erythematous and friable, with punctate ulcerations and mucopus. Skip lesions (intervening normal mucosa within an area of inflammation) are not a feature. Pseudopolyps (**220**), stricture or cancer may be encountered. A colonoscopy may be necessary for defining the extent of the disease. Colonic evaluation is appropriate in all except the most seriously ill patients at risk for toxic megacolon. Nuclear medicine approaches using indium-111- or ^{99m}Tc-labelled autologous leucocytes provide an ability non-invasively to localise colonic inflammation (**215–217, 223**). A timed stool collection and measurement of radioactivity in the stool can provide a quantitative assessment of inflammation.

Complications
Toxic megacolon This is colonic dilatation, with impaired viability of the colonic wall due to secondary bacterial infection, hypoperfusion and stasis; it is a complication of severe colitis (**224**).

224 Toxic megacolon showing grossly dilated colon containing air.

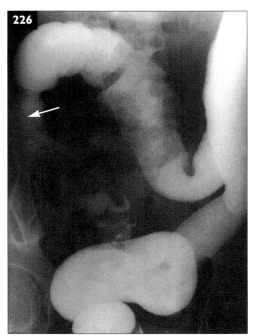

226 Barium X-ray (single contrast) showing a tubular left transverse colon (long-standing ulcerative colitis) and a complicating carcinoma ('apple core' lesion, arrowed) in the ascending colon.

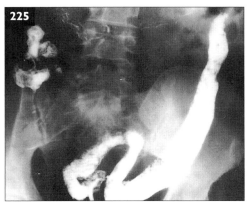

225 Single contrast barium enema showing a tubular featureless left colon of a patient with chronic inflammatory bowel disease.

Ulcerative Colitis

Precipitating factors include hypokalaemia, anti-cholinergic or narcotic drugs, barium enema or air instillation during endoscopy. Early warning signs in plain X-ray are loss of bowel tone with accumulation of gas over long segments of colon, before dilatation occurs. The syndrome of toxic megacolon develops with increased abdominal pain or distension, rebound tenderness, hypo-volaemia, leucocytosis or septic shock. Colonic perforation may be a late feature.

Colon carcinoma This may develop in the setting of long-standing disease (usually >10 years) (**226**, **227**). Mucosal dysplasia in the absence of chronic inflammatory changes is sinister and constitutes a precancerous lesion requiring resection (**221**).

Extraintestinal complications These may be grouped as follows:
• Nutritional and metabolic: protein-losing enteropathy, weight loss and growth retardation, especially in the young.
• Haematological: iron-deficiency anaemia, leucocytosis, thrombocytosis.
• Cutaneous: stomatitis with aphthous ulcers, erythema nodosum, pyoderma gangrenosum (indolent ulcer on extremities with vaso-occlusive features, hyperpigmentation, undermined edges and superinfection of the exudate) (**228**).
• Musculoskeletal: HLA-B27-associated arthro-pathies, such as ankylosing spondylitis (**229**, **230**) or sacroiliitis, arthritis involving peri-pheral large joints, osteoporosis.
• Hepatic: fatty liver, pericholangitis, sclerosing cholangitis, chronic hepatitis, cholangio-carcinoma.
• Renal: nephrolithiasis.
• Ocular: conjunctivitis, episcleritis, iritis, uveitis.
• Obstetric: reduced fertility, increased foetal loss.

Differential diagnosis
Differentiate from Crohn's disease (*Table 4*), infectious proctitis or colitis due to viral, bacterial, fungal or parasitic aetiologies, diverticulitis, radiation colitis, vasculitis, and drug- or toxin-induced enterocolitis.

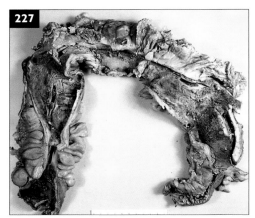

227 Resection specimen of chronic inflammatory bowel disease showing two carcinomas (in right and left colon).

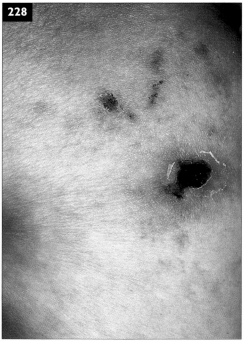

228 Pyoderma gangrenosum, a systemic complication of inflammatory bowel disease.

Ulcerative Colitis

Table 4. Differences between Crohn's disease and ulcerative colitis

	Ulcerative colitis	Crohn's disease
History of smoking	+/–	++
Perianal disease	–	+++
Ileal involvement	–	++
Strictures	+/–	++
Cured by colectomy	+++	–
Endoscopy		
Rectal disease	+++	+
Diffuse and continuous disease	+++	+
Aphthous ulcers	–	+++
Cobblestoning	–	++
Pathology		
Transmural disease	–	+++
Lymphoid aggregates	–	+++
Granulomas	–	++
Fistula	–	+++

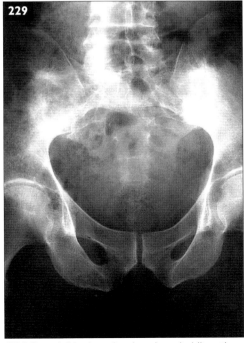

229 Spondylitis; there is sclerosis and obliteration of the normal sacroiliac joint.

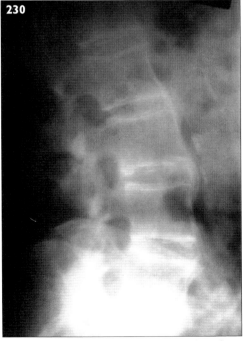

230 'Bamboo spine' – rigid ankylosed spine of ankylosing spondylitis.

Ulcerative Colitis

Prognosis

The course is highly variable, ranging from a single symptomatic episode to recurrent exacerbations or unremitting inflammation and multiple intercurrent complications. Prognosis is determined by the extent and severity of bowel disease, coexisting medical disorders and response to therapies. Toxic megacolon or perforation result in mortality rates of 20–30%. In the elderly, inflammatory bowel disease is not more severe, but outcomes may be worse due to coexisting cardiac, pulmonary or other ailments.

Management

In remission Maintain remission by oral 5-amino salicylates. Salazopyrine, Azulfidine, (sulphapyridine plus 5-ASA) is split by bacteria in the colon to release 5-ASA, but is poorly tolerated in some patients due to nausea, rashes, male infertility and rarely agranulocytosis. Pure 5-ASA preparations (mesalazine) now deliver the drug to the colon without sulphapyridine.

Acute attacks There is some beneficial effect from oral 5-ASA, but additional treatment is generally needed.

Distal disease: requires suppositories, foam or aqueous enemas of 5-ASA or of prednisolone.

Extensive or severe disease: requires systemic steroids, given orally or intravenously. Severe colitis *(Table 3)* is a medical emergency needing admission, intravenous fluids and high-dose parenteral steroids.

Additional immunosuppressive agents, such as 6-mercaptopurine (6-MP), methotrexate, azathioprine and cyclosporine have also been useful for corticosteroid-dependent or - resistant colitis.

Surgery This is necessary for unremitting acute colitis, toxic megacolon and colonic perforation, dysplasia or cancer. The classical surgical procedure of proctocolectomy and ileostomy is now less commonly performed. Sphincter-saving procedures providing continent ileostomies have gained better patient acceptance. The ileo-anal pouch procedure provides for normal rectal passage of stool, although faecal frequency and some faecal seepage are common.

Colonic surveillance by colonoscopy This is necessary at 1- to 2-year intervals to allow detection of dysplasia (**221**) or cancer when colitis is of long duration (≥10 years). When indefinite dysplasia is detected, further surveillance is needed at 3- to 6-month intervals to demonstrate resolution of dysplastic change. In the presence of dysplasia-associated lesion or mass (DALM), colectomy is necessary because the risk of cancer is ≥50%.

Pregnancy tends to exacerbate ulcerative colitis although the risks have been over-emphasised. It is safe to continue sulfasalazine in pregnancy and colitis is usually controlled with corticosteroids.

PROCTITIS

In proctitis, inflammation similarly to that seen in ulcerative colitis may be limited to the lower few centimetres of the rectum. This form probably constitutes about half the cases seen in ambulatory populations. There is often a sharp demarcation between normal and abnormal mucosa. This is now generally thought to be a subtype of ulcerative colitis, and over 10 years, 10–30% of patients experience proximal extension of the inflammation. Treatment is as for ulcerative colitis, but with a greater dependence on local therapies (5-ASA suppositories, local steroids).

Collagenous Colitis/Microscopic Colitis/Lymphocytic Colitis

Definition
Chronic diarrhoea with normal colonic mucosa at endoscopy or radiology, but with chronic mucosal inflammation evident on histology.

Epidemiology and aetiology
The usual age of onset is 60–65 years, and females are much more frequently affected. There may be associated systemic disorders, such as arthritis or autoimmune disorders. The precise aetiology of collagenous colitis or variants is unknown. Some features of colonic injury resemble those produced by non-steroidal anti-inflammatory agents.

Pathophysiology
There is infiltration of the mucosa by a lymphocytic infiltrate. In addition, some patients may have similar inflammatory changes in the small bowel, along with subtotal villous atrophy, which resemble coeliac disease and suggest shared pathogenetic mechanisms. However, unlike coeliac disease, the colonic inflammation does not respond to a gluten-restricted diet. Also, there is no association between collagenous colitis or HLA B8/DR3, which are more prevalent in coeliac disease. Colonic histology is diagnostic. The crypt architecture is preserved, with increased intraepithelial lymphocytes, mildly decreased goblet cells and only rare neutrophils (**231, 232**). Deposition of a layer of type IV collagen in the subepithelial region of the colonic mucosa is most characteristic of collagenous colitis. The band of collagen may be as thick as 100 μm and collagen deposition is most frequent in caecum or transverse colon (>80% of cases) and least in the rectum (<30%). Unlike ulcerative colitis, crypt abscesses are not seen.

Clinical history
Patients report chronic, watery diarrhoea without blood for months or years. Faecal incontinence, nocturnal stools, crampy abdominal pain, nausea and weight loss may be prominent.

Physical examination
There are no specific changes.

Laboratory and special examinations
Typically, expect mild anaemia, hypoalbuminaemia and elevated erythrocyte sedimentation rate. Steatorrhoea is rare. Full colonoscopy is indicated. Multiple colonic biopsies are taken and provide the diagnosis. A rectal biopsy alone is inadequate to exclude the diagnosis.

Differential diagnosis
Differentiate from ulcerative colitis, Crohn's disease, infectious colitis, giardiasis and coeliac disease. The normal endoscopic findings macroscopically are an important diagnostic feature.

Prognosis
No cures are available. The course is variable and the disease usually remains indolent.

Management
Treatment is empiric. Some patients may benefit from cessation of non-steroidal anti-inflammatory agents. Sulfasalazine, 5-ASA and corticosteroids may help in controlling symptoms, but do not reverse collagen deposition.

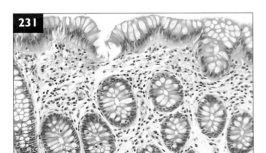 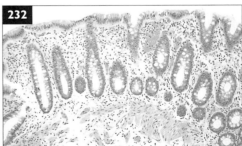

231 & 232 Histopathological appearances of the colon in collagenous colitis (**231**). Note the thick pink area behind the mucosal epithelial layer (collagen). This compares with virtually no pink area in normal colon (**232**).

Radiation Colitis

Definition
Characteristic colonic injury after exposure to ionising radiation, usually manifesting acutely during radiotherapy and also months or years later in an insidious form.

Epidemiology and aetiology
Radiation damage to the bowel usually occurs after exposure to a cumulative dose of 50 Gy (5000 rad). Cells entering DNA synthesis or mitosis are particularly sensitive to radiation injury. External radiation to pelvic organs inevitably exposes portions of the bowel to injury. Brachytherapy (internal radiation with implanted sources) is a safer alternative as the radiation beam is attenuated. The colon is relatively radioresistant, but is most affected by radiation due to the relative immobility of the rectosigmoid region and difficulty in protecting the area while irradiating other organs, especially the prostate.

Pathophysiology
The earliest changes involve microscopic damage to the epithelial cells and vascular endothelial cells, marked submucosal oedema secondary to increased vascular permeability, and superficial ulcerations. In persistent radiation damage, ulceration is extended, vascular endothelium proliferates with telangiectasia, granulation tissue appears, along with atypical fibroblasts and collagen deposition (**233**). Endothelial inflammation and intimal proliferation leads to obliterative arteriopathy. Eventually, the bowel wall atrophies, fibrosis develops and complicating strictures, fistula or leaks occur. Proctosigmoiditis is most common (75%).

Clinical history
Acute radiation proctosigmoiditis presents with diarrhoea, tenesmus and rarely bleeding and usually resolves within 2–6 months. Chronic colitis presents with rectal pain, diarrhoea and bleeding, usually within 2 years of irradiation, but may occur occasionally after decades.

Physical examination
There are no specific abnormalities.

Laboratory and special examinations
Digital rectal examination may be painful. Endoscopy demonstrates pale mucosa, friability and telangiectasia. Discrete ulceration is rare. Endoscopic biopsies usually do not display characteristic features of radiation injury, these usually involve deeper tissues. Barium or gastrograffin enemas may be helpful in demonstrating strictures, fistulas or leaks (**234**).

Differential diagnosis
Differentiate from other colitides, including infectious and ulcerative colitis.

Prognosis
The spontaneous rates of remission are lower in the presence of significant bleeding or anaemia requiring blood transfusion. Surgery is required in ~50% of cases and this may be associated with a greater mortality rate, up to 60%. Recurrent disease is frequent after surgery, and urinary complications are particularly troublesome.

Management
Anti-inflammatory agents, such as sulfasalazine, corticosteroids or sucralfate enemas are tried but usually do not help. Dilatation of strictures may be required. Surgery (resection and reanastomosis or anteroposterior resection) may be required and is often complicated by leaks or sepsis.

Radiation Colitis

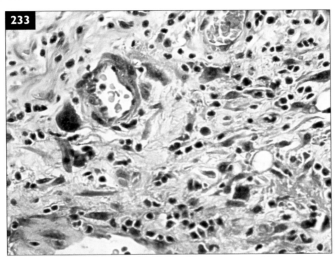

233 Histopathological appearances of radiation enteritis. There are large bizarre fibroblasts showing effects of radiation.

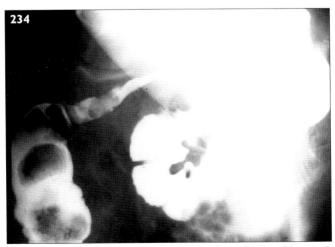

234 Barium enema showing a narrowed stricture in sigmoid caused by radiation.

Infectious Colitis and Proctocolitis

Definition

Infection with bacteria, such as *Shigella*, *Campylobacter* and enteroinvasive or enterohaemorrhagic *E. coli* produces an acute colitis. *Clostridium difficile* infection causes pseudomembranous (**235**) or antibiotic-associated colitis. Acute infectious proctitis may be due to *Chlamydia trachomatis*, *Neisseria gonorrheae*, *Treponema pallidum*, Amoebiasis or herpes simplex type-1.

SHIGELLOSIS

This causes bacillary dysentery due to Shiga exotoxins. Aerobic Gram-negative bacilli fall into four major serotypes: *S. dysenteriae*, *S. boydii*, *S. flexneri* and *S. sonnei*. Transmission is by the faeco-oral route. Shigellosis is prevalent worldwide, with a high attack rate after exposure (60%). The condition is endemic in India, South-East Asia and Mexico. Young children, travellers and institutional residents are most susceptible. Infection is less frequent in developed countries, although ~300 000 cases occur annually in the United States. The incubation period is 1–3 days. Typically, the illness is short-lasting and resolves spontaneously. However, a subacute waxing and waning course lasting 2–3 weeks may be observed. Complications may occur, such as Reiter's syndrome (arthritis, non-specific urethritis and conjunctivitis), as well as ankylosing spondylitis, in HLA-B27 carriers, and rarely haemolytic uraemic syndrome (acute haemolytic anaemia, renal failure and disseminated intravascular coagulation).

CAMPYLOBACTER JEJUNI

This infection is an important cause of bacterial colitis (~20% of cases). The Gram-negative, motile bacteria are transmitted through the oro-faecal route via contaminated poultry, milk, eggs or exposure to sick pets. The incubation period is 1–6 days. Children aged <5 years are most frequently affected. The infection may range from asymptomatic individuals to severe and life-threatening disease with toxic megacolon, pseudomembranous colitis, exacerbation of inflammatory bowel disease and Reiter's syndrome. A relapsing course with rectal bleeding may be seen although stool cultures tend to be negative after 5 weeks in 90% of patients.

ESCHERICHIA COLI

This infection (Gram-negative bacilli) is due to the enteroinvasive *E. coli* (15% of cases) producing 'traveller's diarrhoea' or to the enterohaemorrhagic *E. coli* (O157:H7) strain. Traveller's diarrhoea results from mucosal damage by the invasive bacteria, is usually mild, lasts for 1–3 days and may be prevented by antibiotics, such as doxycycline. The O157:H7 strain causes disease by releasing exotoxins. O157:H7, which may be transmitted by uncooked ground beef (e.g. hamburgers), dairy products or drinking water, causes profuse diarrhoea accompanied by blood after 12–24 hours. Feared complications of haemolytic uraemic syndrome and thrombotic thrombocytopenic purpura may cause fatalities. Several stool cultures may be needed for diagnosis.

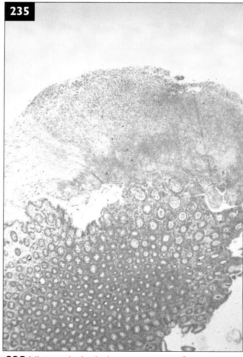

235 Histopathological appearances of pseudomembranous colitis, the pseudomembrane consisting of polymorphonuclear leucocytes.

Infectious Colitis and Proctocolitis

CLOSTRIDIUM DIFFICILE

These Gram-positive bacilli cause disease when the normal bowel flora is altered, such as by antibiotics (particularly penicillins), cancer chemotherapy or another pathogen. The bacteria produce heat-labile exotoxins: toxin A (250 kDa mass) and toxin B (308 kDa), the latter being ~100 times more potent. The toxins are detectable by bio- or immunoassays, both of which are more convenient than culture of the fastidious organism. Occasionally, bacterial toxins may be detected in non-pathogenic settings. The infection is frequently transmitted from infected patients by health-care workers. *C. difficile* infection often complicates inflammatory bowel disease and is responsible for 5–25% of the exacerbations. The manifestations of *C. difficile* infection may range from asymptomatic states, to antibiotic-associated watery diarrhoea and pseudomembranous colitis (**236, 237**). When fulminant, *C. difficile* infection may be life-threatening with marked debilitation, constitutional symptoms, and toxic megacolon, colonic perforation or paralytic ileus.

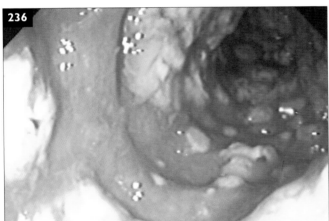

236 Endoscopic appearances of yellow pseudomembranes in *Clostridium difficile* (pseudomembranous colitis).

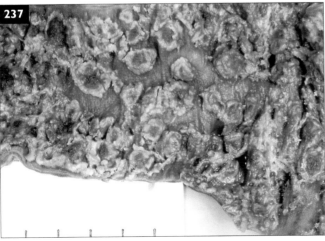

237 Post-mortem specimen of pseudomembranous colitis, showing the circular pseudomembranes.

Infectious Colitis and Proctocolitis

TUBERCULOSIS
Tuberculosis may affect the colon, with *Mycobacterium tuberculosis* of bovine or human strain. The clinical features are those of diarrhoea, pain and bleeding, and have been discussed on page 108. Colonic tuberculosis is diagnosed by a colonoscopy and biopsy with culture, and may be suspected from barium enema findings (**238, 239**).

ACUTE INFECTIOUS PROCTITIS
This condition is usually encountered in the setting of venereal infection in the homosexual or the immunocompromised. Herpetic proctitis is the usual form in the homosexual. The general manifestations of proctitis may accompany more typical features of infection, e.g. inguinal lympha-denopathy in the setting of lymphogranuloma venereum (*Chlamydia trachomatis*), anal canal chancre (syphilis), or anal warts (human papillo-mavirus), although the disease may be localised to the rectum alone, such as in gonorrhoeal proctitis or amoebiasis. Simultaneous evaluation is indicated of the genital organs of the patient and of the contacts (when feasible).

Pathophysiology
The mechanisms common to most infectious colitides involve adhesion of microbes to the bowel wall and epithelial damage due either to the release of exotoxins or to direct cytotoxicity. In comparison with chronic ulcerative colitis, mucin depletion in goblet cells is not as prominent, crypt abscesses are not seen, inflammatory changes tend not to extend to the lamina propria and specific agents, such as viruses or parasites, may be identified. The lesions of pseudomembranous colitis (*C. difficile* infection) are highly characteristic, with prominent outpouring from microulcerated areas in the mucosa of fibrinous exudate containing copious neutrophils (summit lesion) (**235–237**).

Clinical history
The characteristic common features are tenesmus (incomplete sense of bowel evacuation), cramping lower abdominal pain, and small-volume diarrhoea with blood, mucus and leucocytes in the stool. In proctitis, rectal pain is prominent and urinary symptoms, such as retention or poor stream may develop. Fever and constitutional symptoms occur in severe disease. History of antibiotic ingestion in the preceding few weeks or even months (*C. difficile*), homosexual activity (venereal proctitis)

or immunocompromised state (herpes simplex-1 proctitis, amoebiasis, etc.) may be elicited.

Physical examination
Look for fever, tenderness in the left lower quadrant of the abdomen, painful rectal examination with blood, mucus or pus, and possibly features of dehydration.

Laboratory and special examinations
Typically, expect peripheral blood leucocytosis and mild anaemia. Leucocytes in the stool markedly increases the possibility of a positive stool culture. Detection of *C. difficile* toxins in the stool is more convenient than bacterial culture. Sigmoidoscopy reveals erythema, friability, diffuse or typical mucosal ulceration, and exudates or pseudomembranes. Rectal biopsy is diagnostic when characteristic changes are found, e.g. pseudomembranous colitis or cytomegalovirus (**240**), whereas distinction between resolving bacterial and ulcerative colitis may occasionally be difficult. Radiological imaging is helpful only in advanced cases with toxic megacolon or other complications.

Differential diagnosis
Differentiate from inflammatory bowel disease, radiation- or drug-induced colitis, ischaemic colitis and parasitic infestation.

Prognosis
Most patients with infectious colitis make a complete recovery. The onset of acute complications, such as haemolytic uraemic syndrome is associated with poor prognosis, including fatalities. Complications, such as Reiter's syndrome may be associated with a protracted symptomatic course. The most important consequences of infectious colitis involve the public health arena in view of massive worldwide loss of productive activity.

Management
The mainstays are correction of dehydration, contact isolation and prevention of infection in susceptible groups by public health measures. Specific therapeutic interventions are not necessary for all bacterial infections as many resolve by themselves. Shigellosis may be treated by tetracyclines, ampicillin or bactrim, as well as quinolones (ciprofloxacin). *Campylobacter* infections are treated by erythromycin or ciprofloxacin. *E. coli* infections may be treated by

Infectious Colitis and Proctocolitis

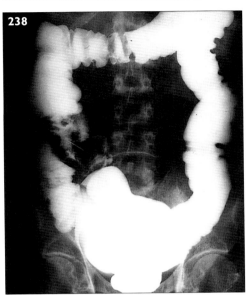

238 A constricted caecum indicated the presence of tuberculosis on this barium enema.

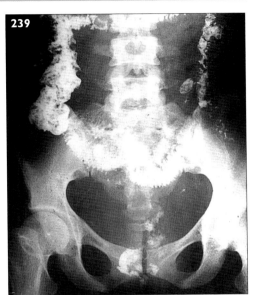

239 Diffuse mucosal thickening and irregularity throughout the colon in this case shows the presence of tuberculous colitis. In addition, the terminal small intestine is abnormal due to lymphangiectasia secondary to tuberculosis.

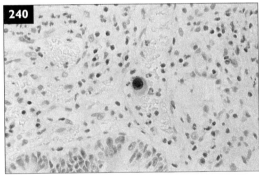

240 A large cell, staining positively for cytomegalovirus antibodies, in a patient with cytomegalovirus colitis.

bactrim, ampicillin, quinolones and tetracycline. *C. difficile* infection requires antibiotic treatment. Although more expensive, oral vancomycin may show a slightly greater efficacy (~90–95%) than either oral or intravenous metronidazole (85–90%). Relapses of *C. difficile* infection may require repeat courses of the same antibiotic or a switch to the other, and if the relapse is after initial treatment with metronidazole, it is generally accepted that vancomycin should be substituted. Alternative agents for treating *C. difficile* infection are bacitracin and teicoplanin. Lymphogranuloma

venereum is treated by tetracycline, gonorrhoea and syphilis by penicillin or cephalosporins, HSV-1 by acyclovir and human papillomavirus (HPV) by podophyllin or cryotherapy.

ACTINOMYCOSIS

This is a chronic invasive fungus with a propensity for the ileocaecal region, and which causes mass, local fistulae and perforation. It is generally only diagnosed at laparotomy. The differential diagnosis is appendix mass, Crohn's disease, lymphoma or carcinoma of the caecum.

Drug and Chemical Colitis

Definition
This condition is defined as colitis resulting from the direct actions of soaps, water-soluble contrast media, hydrogen peroxide, acids, alkali, irritants, and laxatives or other agents. Mild injury not coming to medical attention may be far more frequent than severe injury. The public interest in 'colonic lavage' for improving health and the incorporation of untested, exotic ingredients into cleansing enemas may enhance the overall incidence of injury. Mild inflammation is common, but severe acute colitis, perforation and cicatrisation over 3–4 weeks may be seen.

MELANOSIS COLI
This refers to dark pigmentation of the colonic mucosa (241) with a reticulated appearance after exposure to anthraquinone laxatives (cascara, aloe, rhubarb, senna, frangula, etc.).

Epidemiology, aetiology and pathophysiology
Melanosis is due to the deposition of brown, granular pigment consisting of melanin or lipofuscin within macrophages in the lamina propria. The number of macrophages increases between colonic crypts with epithelial cells demonstrating apoptosis, as well as ultrastructural abnormalities of uncertain significance. Colonic melanosis requires a mean of nine months to develop but may occur within four months and resolves upon discontinuation of the incriminating agent. The overall prevalence is 0.25–24% of colonoscopies. Patients are typically aged >40 years and female. The caecum and rectum are commonly affected, although the entire colon may be involved.

Clinical history
There are no specific symptoms.

Physical examination
There are no systemic or peripheral abnormalities.

Laboratory and special examinations
Endoscopy and biopsy are diagnostic. The colonic mucosa appears black or slate grey with reticulated striations or spots reminiscent of alligator skin.

Differential diagnosis
None.

Prognosis
This is a benign disorder. No greater cancer risk has been identified.

Management
By removal of the incriminant.

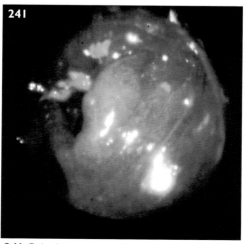

241 Colonic appearance in melanosis coli reflecting laxative abuse.

Cathartic Colon

Definition
Defined as colonic sequelae of chronic laxative abuse.

Epidemiology and aetiology
The manifestations are related to persistent and excessive use of laxatives, such as anthraquinones. Patients may suffer from chronic constipation, preoccupation with bowel movements, psychological disturbances or surreptitious drug use.

Pathophysiology
Persistent and excessive laxative intake damages the myenteric neural plexus with colonic dysmotility, as well as causing gross morphological alterations. The resulting rapid transit through the bowel may occasionally even manifest with impaired digestion (steatorrhoea or excess protein loss via the stool).

Clinical history
Typically, there is abdominal bloating or fullness, lower abdominal cramping pain, and diarrhoea or constipation. A history of excess laxative intake may not readily be elicited.

Physical examination
No specific examination is suggested.

Laboratory and special examinations
Look for serum electrolyte abnormalities, such as hypokalaemia. A plain radiograph or barium enema demonstrates characteristic features, such as loss of haustra, foreshortening and conical shape of the caecum, and dilatation of the colon into a tubular shape (242, 243). Biopsies are usually normal. Melanosis coli may be an accompaniment, but not necessarily so. If laxative abuse is denied, chemical identification of laxatives in the urine may be helpful (244).

Differential diagnosis
Some morphological features may superficially resemble chronic ulcerative colitis, but the distinction is usually straightforward.

Prognosis
Resolution depends upon the ability to discontinue laxatives. Most changes resolve within a few months.

Management
Withdrawal of laxatives is most important. This usually requires bowel retraining, the use of bulking agents, and switching to osmotic laxatives or enemas. In refractory cases, recourse to drastic measures, such as total or subtotal colectomy may be required.

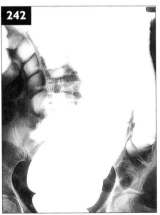

242 Megacolon, reflecting long-term laxative abuse.

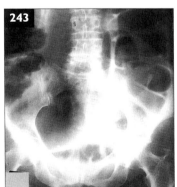

243 Gross colonic dilatation seen in a patient with megacolon due to laxatives. The maintenance of a normal haustral pattern differentiates this from toxic megacolon.

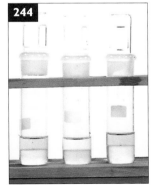

244 A positive anthracene test showing the presence of senna or one of its derivatives in a patient abusing laxative.

Parasitic Infestations of the Colon

Definition

Amoebiasis, schistosomiasis and Chagas' disease are most remarkable for involvement of the colon, as well as other organs. Pinworm or whipworm infestations also are frequent.

AMOEBIASIS

The causative agent is *Entamoeba histolytica* (EH). A variety of saprophytic entamoebas, which only rarely cause disease, colonise humans and a distinction must be made between these and the pathogenic *E. histolytica*.

Epidemiology and aetiology

After malaria and schistosomiasis, amoebiasis is the most prevalent parasitic disease in the world, accounting annually for >500 million cases, with colitis or liver abscess in ~50 million and death in ~100 000 people. The greatest prevalence is in India, Africa and central and south America. The groups at greatest risk are inhabitants of, or immigrants from, endemic areas, promiscuous male homosexuals, and the institutionalised.

Pathophysiology

The virulence depends upon the EH strain, as well as interactions with colonic bacteria, and host-specific factors. After oro-faecal transmission of EH cysts, trophozoites arise through excystation and adhere to the colonic epithelium. The trophozoites release proteases and collagenases, as well as endotoxins, which result in mucosal inflammation, lysis and a host immune response. The trophozoites may travel to the liver via the portal vein, producing an abscess (**245**). Exposure to EH generates long-lasting antibodies against surface antigens of the parasite, as well as T-lymphocyte responses that decrease recurrence of disease; e.g. a second amoebic liver abscess is highly unusual (<3 cases/1000).

Clinical history

Symptoms vary widely, depending upon the extent and nature of colonisation, and include asymptomatic cyst-carriers, which constitute reservoirs of infection. Manifestations include diarrhoea, acute amoebic dysentery (proctocolitis with blood and mucus in the stool), chronic non-dysenteric amoebiasis (diarrhoea, mucus weight loss and colonic ulceration), amoeboma (localised mass of granulation tissue), toxic megacolon, colonic stricture or amoebic peritonitis. Extraintestinal manifestations include liver abscess (10%) and cutaneous or venereal amoebiasis. Hepatic abscesses may rupture into contiguous organs, such as the lung, pericardium and inferior vena cava.

Physical examination

Weight loss, fever and dehydration. Tender hepatomegaly, upper abdominal distension, haematochezia and leucocytes in the stool. Jaundice or peritonitis are uncommon.

Laboratory and special examinations

Typically, expect leucocytosis, anaemia, hypoalbuminaemia, elevated serum alkaline phosphatase and elevated prothrombin time. Prepare wet stool preparations (×3) (**246**) or endoscopic stool smears for trophozoites. Colonoscopy (without enemas or laxatives for preparation) shows haemorrhagic mucosa and discrete ulcers, typically with a shallow base and raised, undermined edges. The disease may be limited to the rectum, caecum or ascending colon. Biopsies from the edge of the ulcers may demonstrate EH (periodic acid–Schiff stain). The anti-amoebic antibody is of diagnostic value in amoebic liver abscess (sensitivity, 99%) or amoebic dysentery (sensitivity, 88%) but does not distinguish between previous or active infection. Imaging modalities (ultrasound/CT/MRI/^{99m}Tc-liver scan) are helpful in identifying liver abscess.

Differential diagnosis

Differentiate from inflammatory bowel disease, irritable colon syndrome, colitis due to other causes or pyogenic liver abscess.

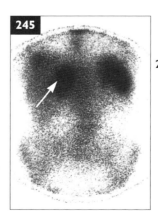

245 This white cell scan shows (arrow) localisation of white cells within the liver. This shows the presence of a liver abscess secondary to portal pyaemia.

Parasitic Infestations of the Colon

Prognosis
Fulminant colitis or liver abscess may prove fatal (**247**). Amoebiasis is most severe in the malnourished, young, elderly, pregnant, or immunosuppressed (20–30% case fatality rates).

Management
Invasive colonic disease and liver abscess are treated by metronidazole for 10 days. Liver abscess may also be treated by a combination of metronidazole and chloroquine. More toxic drugs include emetine and dihydroemetine. Percutaneous aspiration is necessary only for liver abscesses with impending rupture. Surgery is rarely indicated. Asymptomatic cyst passers may be treated by diloxanide furoate, iodoquinol or paromomycin, although reinfection is frequent in endemic areas.

SCHISTOSOMIASIS
Epidemiology and aetiology
Schistosomiasis (*Schistosoma mansoni*) is widespread in Africa, Latin America and the Middle-East. *Schistosoma japonicum* is prevalent in the Far East, including China, Japan, Philippines and Indo-China. Humans serve as the definitive host. The ova are excreted in the stools and hatch into miracidia upon reaching fresh water. Further development into cercariae occurs in freshwater snails. Through human water-related activities, cercaria gain access to the skin, enter the body and mature into adult worms in the superior mesenteric vein (*S. mansoni*) or inferior mesenteric vein (*S. japonicum*). *S. haematobium* live in the vesical plexus and only rarely cause gastrointestinal complications. The worms live their life as pairs, with the female living inside the male within venules and release 300–3500 eggs daily. Lytic enzymes produced by the ova facilitate penetration by the worm of the venule wall and entry into the intestinal lumen.

Pathophysiology
The cutaneous migration of larvae excites local inflammation (cutaneous larva migrans). Deposition of ova into the portal vein or the intestinal wall leads to chronic inflammation and fibrosis. The eventual consequences depend upon the worm burden, as well as the host immune response.

Clinical history
Cutaneous larva migrans may be asymptomatic or excite mild pruritic dermatitis. Visceral larva migrans may be associated with fever, urticaria,

serum sickness-like illness, cough, weight loss and eosinophilia. Colonic schistosomiasis may cause abdominal pain, diarrhoea and blood in the stool. Strictures (**248**) or polyps may occur. Periportal

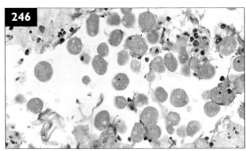

246 Stool examination shows the presence of round amoebae, which have ingested red cells, showing that they are pathogenic.

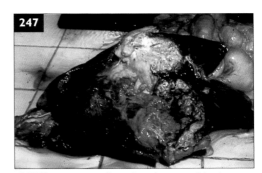

247 Post-mortem liver showing amoebic abscess.

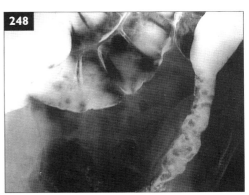

248 Narrowed irregular colonic appearances in a patient with schistosomiasis on barium enema.

Parasitic Infestations of the Colon

liver fibrosis causes portal hypertension, hepatosplenomegaly, variceal bleeding and ascites with a relatively preserved hepatic parenchymal function. Portasystemic shunting of eggs to the lungs may cause chronic pulmonary hypertension and cor pulmonale.

Physical examination
Typical findings in advanced cases are hepatosplenomegaly, ascites or prominent abdominal collateral veins. Early cases may show no abnormal signs.

Laboratory and special examinations
Investigations are for ova in the stool (**249**), and rectal or liver biopsy (**250**). Direct smears have a low sensitivity. Colonoscopy may demonstrate diffuse or patchy erythema, friability and 'schistosomal polyps' containing eggs and granulation tissue. Serologic tests may be suggestive, but are not diagnostic.

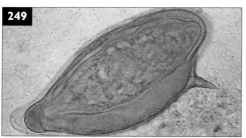

249 Stool examination showing the presence of a schistosome, the laterally placed spike shows that it is S. mansoni.

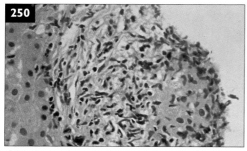

250 A granuloma in the liver of a patient with schistosomiasis.

Differential diagnosis
Differentiate from other causes of portal hypertension, diarrhoea, abdominal pain and rectal bleeding.

Prognosis
The course is indolent and eradication of the worms has generally been difficult. Co-infection with either hepatitis B or C virus markedly accelerates liver disease. If fatal, patients usually die of liver disease.

Management
Praziquantel kills the worms and is indicated for all patients. Oxamniquine is an alternative for *S. mansoni*. However, eradication of the worms may not reverse the disease. Symptomatic treatments are necessary for gastrointestinal bleeding, ascites and heart failure. The development of a vaccine is being actively pursued.

CHAGAS' DISEASE (*TRYPANOSOMA CRUZI*) EPIDEMIOLOGY AND AETIOLOGY
Chagas' disease afflicts millions in Latin America with thousands of deaths annually. The parasite is transmitted from infected humans or animals with circulating trypomastigotes by the reduvid bug. Metacyclic trypomastigotes develop in the insect intestines and enter humans through contamination of insect bites with insect faeces containing infectious trypomastigotes.

Pathophysiology
The host genetics, parasite factors and autoimmune responses involved in disease pathogenesis are incompletely defined. Myocardial destruction and fibrosis is characteristic and the myenteric plexus in the gastrointestinal tract is destroyed with abnormal gut hormone responses.

Clinical history
Acute infections are usually asymptomatic, although periorbital oedema at the site of the reduvid bug bite, fever, adenopathy, hepatosplenomegaly or myocarditis may be noted. Chronic infection manifests years later with cardiac or gastrointestinal disease. Cardiac arrhythmias, cardiomyopathy, dysphagia, regurgitation and constipation are typical.

Physical examination
Look for cardiomegaly, megaoesophagus and megacolon.

Parasitic Infestations of the Colon

Laboratory and special examinations
Take Giemsa-stained smears from tissues, cultivation of organisms in special media and serologic tests. Analysis of reduvid bugs may help. Chest radiograph, plain radiograph of abdomen and barium studies of the oesophagus and colon are helpful.

Differential diagnosis
Differentiate from a variety of gastrointestinal disorders causing neuromuscular disease, including myopathies, autonomic neuropathy, progressive systemic sclerosis, Hirschsprung's disease, drug-induced pseudo-obstruction (narcotics, laxative abuse, antidepressants, etc.).

Prognosis
The natural history is of progressive deterioration and death due to cardiac complications.

Management
Only symptomatic treatments are available. Specific therapies are under development.

ENTEROBIUS VERMICULARIS (PINWORM)
Epidemiology and aetiology
This is a parasitic worm endemic in temperate and tropical climates. Schoolchildren are most frequently affected. Poor personal hygiene is usually incriminated. The transmission is by ingestion of ova, which hatch in the upper small bowel and mature during transit through the ileum. The adult worms live in the distal colon.

Pathophysiology
The female migrates through the anus to lay eggs in perianal or perineal skin, which leads to local symptoms.

Clinical history
If symptomatic, there is perianal skin irritation, pruritus ani, vulvovaginitis, and occasionally granulomatous peritonitis (migration of worms through the colonic wall or female genital tract).

Physical examination
Perianal erythema or secondary infection.

Laboratory and special examinations
This is by microscopic examination of worms picked up on adhesive cellophane tape applied to the anal region (sensitivity of three smears, 90%). Identification of stool ova and parasites is less sensitive (10–15%).

Differential diagnosis
Differentiate from other worm infections.

Prognosis
Worm eradication requires improved personal hygiene, treatment of other family members and thorough decontamination of bed-linen and personal clothing.

Management
Mebendazole, albendazole or pyrantel pamoate are effective wormicidal agents.

TRICHURIS TRICHURIA (WHIPWORM)
Epidemiology and aetiology
This parasite is prevalent in the tropics. Infection occurs by contact with contaminated stool. After ingestion of embryonated eggs, the larvae excyst and penetrate the intestinal mucosa with their thread-like anterior ends, moult, mature and reattach as adults to the caecal or colonic mucosa. The mature females release 2000–6000 eggs daily. The maturation of eggs requires 10–14 days in the soil.

Pathophysiology
Symptoms depend upon the worm burden and are due to mechanical or parasitic phenomena. Children are most commonly affected.

Clinical history
Presentation ranges from asymptomatic states to anaemia, growth retardation, and bloody or mucoid stools. Rectal prolapse and colonic obstruction or perforation are rare.

Physical examination
This is not helpful.

Laboratory and special examinations
Monitor eosinophilia, ova in the stools, and worms in the colonic mucosa.

Differential diagnosis
Differentiate from other parasitic infestations.

Prognosis
Usually excellent.

Management
Worms are eradicated by mebendazole or albendazole. In addition, public health measures should be taken (sanitary stool disposal, hand washing, proper cleaning and cooking of food).

Diverticular Disease of the Colon

Definition
Colonic diverticula represent bowel wall projections that create extraluminal pouches. Diverticulitis results from inflammatory exacerbations due to impacted materials in the diverticula.

Epidemiology and aetiology
The prevalence is far greater in industrialised societies, particularly in the west. Diverticula are rarely observed before 40 years of age, ranging between 5–45% of cases overall. There is an age-dependent increase in the prevalence of colonic diverticula, which may exceed 50% in people aged over 80 years. In Western societies, differences in dietary fibre intake and switching to low-residue diets are believed to account for increased prevalence. Diverticular disease is rare in agrarian societies with high dietary fibre intake, such as in Africa and India. Whether additional host-specific factors contribute is unclear.

Pathophysiology
The diverticula arise in the colon where colonic arteries penetrate the muscularis to reach the mucosa (251). The diverticula lack muscularis mucosa and are of pulsion type, probably related to prolonged straining at stool and excessively increased intracolonic pressures. Diverticula are mostly in the sigmoid and the left-sided colon (95%), less frequently in the ascending, transverse and descending colon (35%) and least often throughout the colon (7%). Diverticulitis develops when the mouth of a diverticulum becomes impacted by faecal material, followed by erosion through the serosa, leakage or perforation, and development of an inflammatory mass. Erosion into a blood vessel may produce profuse haemorrhage, although this is uncommon.

Clinical history
Most cases are asymptomatic (70%). Diverticulitis (10–25%) presents with subacute left lower quadrant pain, fever and constipation or loose stools. Rectal haemorrhage (5%) is infrequent.

Physical examination
Typically, tachycardia, fever and tenderness, distension or mass in the left lower quadrant in the presence of diverticulitis. In the absence of complications there are no abnormal signs.

Laboratory and special examinations
Laboratory findings include leucocytosis and mild anaemia. A plain radiograph of the abdomen may demonstrate air beneath the

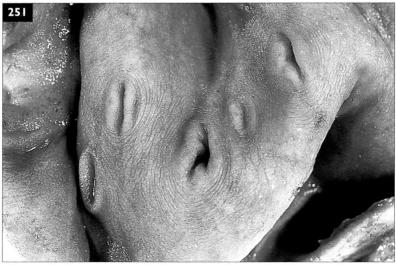

251 A resection specimen showing colonic diverticula from the luminal side.

Diverticular Disease of the Colon

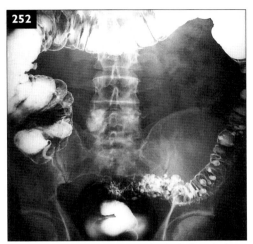

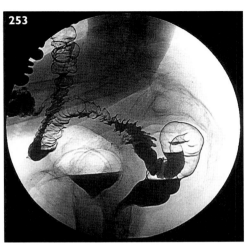

252 Barium enema showing classical diverticular disease predominantly in the sigmoid and descending colon, though scattered diverticula are present on the right-hand side. (Some barium is also seen in the bladder, indicating a colo-vesical fistula.)

253 Complicated diverticular disease, with a fistula well demonstrated between the sigmoid colon and the bladder.

diaphragm or extraluminal gas if bowel perforation has occurred. A barium enema may demonstrate mucosal irregularities and bowel spasm, perforation, abscess or fistula formation (**252, 253**). A colonoscopy may be helpful in distinguishing from colitis or cancer (**254**). CT is useful for assessing bowel thickening and abscess formation.

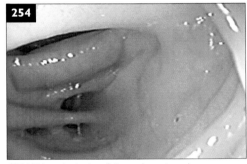

254 Diverticulosis of the colon at endoscopy.

Differential diagnosis
Differentiate from inflammatory bowel disease, bacterial colitis, ischaemic bowel disease, irritable colon syndrome, colon cancer, gynaecological disorders, e.g. salpingo-oophoritis. Remember that diverticulosis is common and may coexist with these conditions.

Prognosis
Patients may remain asymptomatic throughout life or have only minimal symptoms. Severe diverticulitis may require surgical intervention. Bleeding may be paroxysmal and life-threatening. Complications include colonic stricture, perforation, abscess and fistulous communications with adjacent organs, including urinary bladder and small intestine, and septicaemia.

Management
Diverticulitis is treated with antibiotics (third-generation cephalosporin plus metronidazole), intravenous fluids and bowel rest for several days. Abscesses may be drained percutaneously. Unremitting disease may require surgical intervention and hemicolectomy, debridement or additional measures. Increased dietary fibre intake, stool softeners and avoidance of constipation help in decreasing symptoms of diverticular disease.

Hirschsprung's Disease and Congenital Megacolon

Definition
A developmental disorder characterised by defective neural crest cell migration during colonic development leading to an 'aganglionic' segment.

Epidemiology and aetiology
Genetic mutations have been identified with autosomal recessive (chromosome 13) and autosomal dominant (chromosome 10) transmission. The disorder is relatively uncommon and may come to diagnosis in neonates, early childhood or adult life.

Pathophysiology
The aganglionic segment of the colon causes a functional obstruction due to a failure to relax. The proximal bowel is hypertrophied and dilated. The rectosigmoid region is most frequently affected (75–80%), although the entire colon and variable lengths of the small bowel may be affected (5–10%). The affected segment is usually very short in adults.

Clinical history
• In the new-born: there is delayed passage of meconium and abdominal distension.
• In children: there is chronic constipation, abdominal distension, volvulus or perforation.
• In adults: there is chronic constipation from childhood or dramatic intermittent constipation.

Physical examination
A rectal examination shows an empty rectal vault in Hirschsprung's disease, whereas stool is present in idiopathic megacolon.

Laboratory and special examinations
Plain radiograph of the abdomen shows colonic dilatation and a paucity of gas in the rectum. A barium enema shows a short, narrow segment or transition zone (255) and may be normal. Anal manometry demonstrates failure of the internal sphincter to relax in response to rectal distension. Histology using a full-thickness biopsy is usually necessary for diagnosis. The most typical feature is absence of ganglion cells in the submucosa and myenteric plexus, identification of which is facilitated by acetylcholinesterase staining.

Differential diagnosis
Differentiate from other structural and congenital abnormalities (intestinal duplications, malrotation, imperforate anus, volvulus), Chagas' disease, other causes of colonic dilatation.

Prognosis
This is usually good.

Management
Treatment is surgical. Neonates may require a colostomy or pull-through of the bowel to the anus. In short-segment aganglionosis, rectal myectomy alone may be adequate.

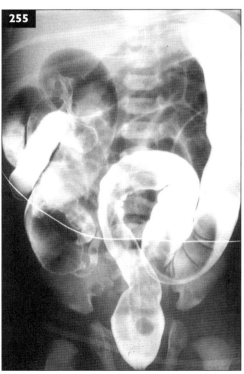

255 Barium enema in Hirschprung's disease in a newborn, showing a short, narrow segment or transition zone and dilated colon above.

Solitary Rectal Ulcer

Definition
Non-specific ulceration of the rectum with characteristic disorganisation of the muscularis mucosa.

Epidemiology and aetiology
The disorder is infrequent and tends to affect young adults, females more than males, usually in the third or the fourth decade of life, although the age range is wider (10–80 years). Chronic constipation and straining at stool, as well as rectal injury during manual stool evacuation may be involved.

Pathophysiology
The precise chain of events has not been reproduced. It is thought that straining and excessive voiding pressure during stool evacuation may produce rectal prolapse, functional ischaemia and ulceration. Local trauma may play a role.

Clinical history
Constipation, tenesmus, straining at stool and lower abdominal pain are frequent (70–90%). Mild rectal bleeding may occur (50–90% of cases) but profuse rectal bleeding is highly unusual. One-quarter of the patients are asymptomatic.

Physical examination
Rectal induration or bleeding may be apparent on digital examination. The ulcers are usually within a few centimetres of the anal verge and may affect the anterior or the posterior rectal wall.

Laboratory and special examinations
Iron-deficiency anaemia may be found. Unless carefully sought, the ulcers may be missed on flexible sigmoidoscopy (256). In view of their distal location, proctoscopy may be superior in visualisation of a solitary rectal ulcer. Ulcers are shallow, but with an indurated edge. Biopsies from the edge of the ulcer demonstrate replacement of the lamina propria by fibroblasts, smooth muscle and collagen. There is associated hypertrophy and disorganisation of the muscularis mucosa, displacement of mucosal glands into the submucosa and mucosal ulceration. The diffuse infiltration with collagen fibres is characteristic.

Differential diagnosis
Differentiate from Crohn's disease, ulcerative colitis, chronic ischaemic colitis, malignancy, venereal disease and amoebiasis.

Prognosis
This is usually good.

Management
The mainstays are bulk laxatives, bowel retraining and patient education. In refractory cases or with excessive bleeding, local excision, rectopexy or (rarely) diverting colostomy may be performed.

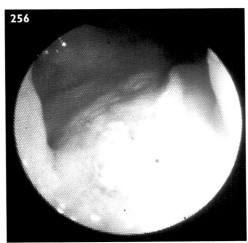

256 A solitary rectal ulcer seen on colonoscopy.

Vascular Disorders of the Colon

Obliteration of the colonic blood flow results in ischaemic injury. The vascular process affecting the coeliac axis, superior mesenteric or inferior mesenteric circulation may be occlusive, non-occlusive, or a combination of these. Whether the colon suffers ischaemic damage depends upon the state of the general circulation, collateral blood flow, response to autonomic stimuli, release of circulating vasoactive substances and local modulation of blood flow. Disease occurs most frequently from colonic ischaemia (60%) or acute mesenteric ischaemia affecting the small intestine (30%) and less often from chronic mesenteric ischaemia (5%) or focal segmental ischaemia (5%). Colonic angiodysplasia, telangiectasia or portasystemic varices constitute additional vascular disorders.

ISCHAEMIC COLITIS
Definition
Colonic injury due to interrupted blood supply.

Epidemiology and aetiology
The colon may be affected by superior mesenteric artery disease (50% occlusion, 25% ischaemia, 10% thrombosis) in the setting of left atrial or ventricular thrombosis, acute myocardial infarction, congestive heart failure, arrhythmias and shock; thrombosis of the superior mesenteric vein due to hypercoagulative states, coagulation disorders, polycythemia vera or oestrogen excess; and by focal segmental ischaemia (10%) from emboli, vasculitis, radiation, trauma, intestinal obstruction, enteritis, hernia, etc. Isolated colonic ischaemia mostly affects patients aged over 60 years (90%) and in this setting no apparent cause may be found at presentation. Younger individuals may present with colonic injury due to vasculitis, sickle cell disease, coagulopathies, drugs – such as cocaine – and, occasionally, long-distance running.

Pathophysiology
Simultaneous involvement of the small and large gut in ischaemic injury (coeliac or superior mesenteric artery occlusion) is devastating, with mortality rates approaching 90% in the presence of peritonitis. Involvement of the colon alone most frequently causes reversible submucosal or intramural haemorrhage (30–40%), transient necrosis (15–20%), gangrene (15–20%), chronic ulceration (20–25%), or stricture (10–15%), and less often fulminant necrosis (~5%). The systemic manifestations are related to perfusion–reperfusion injury and release of vasoactive substances or inflammatory mediators. The histological correlates of acute ischaemic colitis are extensive haemorrhage, congestion, oedema (**257**) and necrosis (**258**) with or without perforation, gangrene and stricture. Although any part of the colon may be affected, the splenic flexure, descending colon and sigmoid colon are most often involved in acute ischaemic colitis.

Clinical history
There is sudden cramping left lower abdominal pain, tenesmus and bright red or maroon blood per rectum. Acute mesenteric ischaemia may be 'silent' and patients can present with shock, confusion or metabolic acidosis.

Physical examination
Typically, there are diminished or absent bowel sounds, lower abdominal tenderness and signs of peritonitis or bowel perforation.

Laboratory and special examinations
Expect leucocytosis, anaemia, metabolic acidosis, elevated serum amylase, lactate dehydrogenase and creatine phosphokinase. A plain radiograph of the abdomen may show colonic intramural oedema or haemorrhage producing 'thumb-printing', as well as free air in the peritoneal cavity. Colonoscopy or flexible sigmoidoscopy may show extensive mucosal haemorrhage and congestion (**259**). A barium enema may interfere with subsequent angiography. Visceral angiography can demonstrate the site of occlusion.

Differential diagnosis
Differentiate from inflammatory bowel disease, infectious colitis, radiation colitis and the various causes of acute abdomen.

Prognosis
Acute mesenteric ischaemia is fatal in 40–50% of cases, with mortality rates approaching 90% in the presence of generalised peritonitis (indicating bowel perforation). In isolated colonic involvement, the prognosis is better with only submucosal or intramural haemorrhage in two-thirds and transient colitis in one-third. Irreversible colonic injury occurs in 50% of cases, however. Patients may re-present with a delayed stricture 4–6 weeks after an initial acute presentation with diarrhoea and bleeding.

Vascular Disorders of the Colon

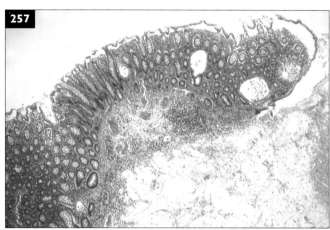

257 Histopathological section showing swollen congested mucosa with loss of epithelial cells in ischaemic colitis.

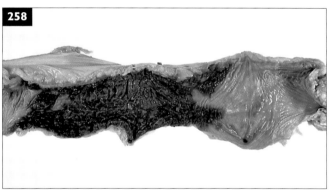

258 A localised area of necrotic colon. This is a resection specimen from a patient with ischaemic colitis.

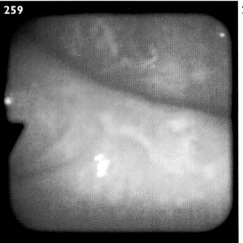

259 Endoscopic appearances of the splenic flexure showing congestion in ischaemic colitis.

Vascular Disorders of the Colon

Management
Patients with severe disease require aggressive resuscitation and intensive care, broad-spectrum antibiotics and surgery. In the absence of perforation or gangrene, patients may be managed by bowel rest and antibiotics.

COLONIC ANGIODYSPLASIA
Definition
Vascular ectasias affecting the colonic mucosa in the absence of cutaneous lesions, systemic disease or a familial syndrome.

Epidemiology and aetiology
Prospective studies are necessary to determine the true prevalence. Asymptomatic angio-dysplasia is frequent and may be found in 3–6% of cases at colonoscopy. Angiodysplasia is one of the most common causes of recurrent gastrointestinal bleeding in the elderly. Most patients with symptoms are aged over 70 years, although patients may present earlier. There is a loosely defined association of uncertain significance between colonic angiodysplasia and valvular aortic stenosis.

Pathophysiology
Angiodysplasia is most common in the caecum and ascending colon. Prominent dilated and tortuous submucosal veins are the earliest and most constant feature of angiodysplasia (260, 261). The ectasias consist of dilated, thin-walled distorted veins, venules or capillaries lined by epithelium alone, or by variable amounts of smooth muscle. Most ectasias are <1 cm in diameter. More than one ectatic lesions are generally found.

Clinical history
Recurrent rectal blood loss in the elderly with bright red or maroon-coloured blood. Massive bleeding is uncommon (<15% of cases). Bleeding tends to stop by itself (90%). Anaemia due to chronic occult bleeding may be the presenting manifestation. Other more florid angiomatous malformations (262) may give a similar clinical picture.

Physical examination
Typical findings are anaemia, cardiac lesions and atherosclerotic peripheral vascular disease in some cases.

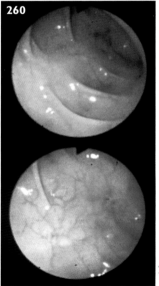

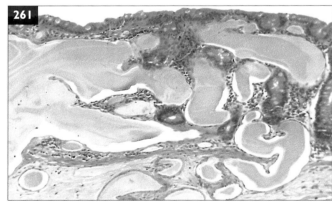

261 Injected histopathological specimen (light-pink injectate) showing dilated vascular spaces in the submucosa in caecal angiodysplasia.

260 Angiodysplasia of the caecum showing red spider-like vascular anomalies.

Vascular Disorders of the Colon

Laboratory and special examinations
Look for iron-deficiency anaemia. Colonoscopy by the inexperienced may lead to overdiagnosis of angiodysplasia (sensitivity >80%). Total colonoscopy with good visualisation of the caecum is necessary to exclude angiodysplasia. Angiography (**263**) is diagnostic when one of the following is seen: dilated and slowly emptying vein within the bowel wall, arterial 'tufting' pattern, or an early filling vein during the arterial phase. Identification of the lesions in pathology specimens requires special techniques, such as instillation of barium or polymers in the vessels.

Differential diagnosis
Differentiate from malignancy, diverticular disease and ischaemic colitis.

Prognosis
The course is usually indolent. Many patients remain asymptomatic throughout life. Bleeding may continue after 1–2 years in only 50% of patients.

Management
Treatment is usually conservative in view of advanced age, associated disorders and rebleeding only in some patients. Endoscopic ablation of lesions by cautery, heat or laser is often successful. The lesions can also be controlled by angiographic embolisation. Surgical resection may be necessary. Oestrogen–progesterone combinations have occasionally been beneficial.

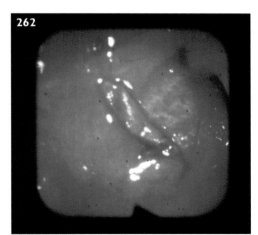

262 Endoscopic appearances of colonic haemangioma.

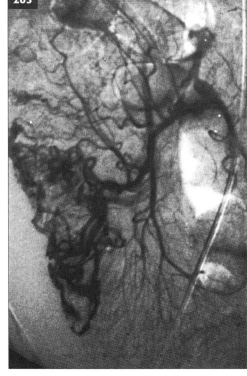

263 Visceral angiogram (arterial phase) showing increased vascularity in the caecum (much denser than in the ascending colon) and early filling of the venous phase from that area.

Haemorrhoids, Anal Fissures and Fistulae

The venous plexus of vessels around the anorectal junction helps form a mucosal-covered cushion that aids continence. Haemorrhoids (piles in the vernacular) develop from congestion of venous plexuses, with associated mucosal hypertrophy and development of adjacent perirectal skin tags (264). In the more severe cases, parts of the venous plexus with the overlying mucosa prolapse from the rectum.

Symptoms
Various symptoms are identified. Perianal itching may be associated with haemorrhoids; bleeding is the most common symptom leading to seeking medical attention. Characteristically, there is bright red on the surface of the stool and on the lavatory paper, and not mixed with the stools. Thrombosis of external piles leads to a painful hard round lesion.

Management
Avoidance measures Prevention of straining at stool, passage of soft stool.

Treatment Maintenance of bowel habit as above. Bleeding may be treated by local sclerosis, or larger piles by ligation and banding surgically. Anal dilatation (under anaesthesia) may be used.

ACUTE ANAL FISSURES
This appears as a split in the surface epithelium of the anorectal junction, and causes substantial pain, particularly during defaecation. It is particularly likely to occur with severe constipation.

Management
Two approaches are possible: treating the constipation to allow regular passage of soft stool (as internal dilator); a high fibre intake helps. In the short term, dilatation of the rectum will allow stretching of the anal rectal sphincter, and can initiate healing of the mucosa.

ANAL FISTULA
Perianal fistula
Fistulous tracks may develop from the anal canal or the rectum, commencing as sinuses and tracking into the perianal tissue, and in some instances opening out on to the perianal skin. Infection within these fistulous tracks causes both abscesses and persistent discharge from fistulous openings. Low fistulae open below the internal anal sphincter, and high fistulae open above. Complex fistulae are often associated with

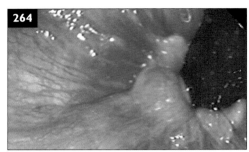

264 Retroflexed view in the rectum showing normal rectal mucosa, but haemorrhoids around the anal margin.

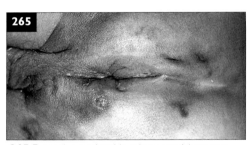

265 Extensive perianal involvement (abscesses and fistulae) in Crohn's disease.

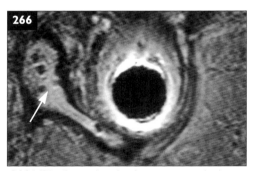

266 MRI using anal probe (transverse section) demonstrating (arrowed) a perianal fistula and perianal abscess formation.

Crohn's disease (265). MRI can allow fistulous tracts to be imaged in great detail (266). The symptoms are those of pain and discharge, and treatment varies from antibiotics alone, release of pus under pressure and, in persistent cases, local surgical treatment to lay fistulae open and allow healing with obliteration of the tract.

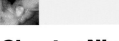

Chapter Nine

Gastrointestinal Bleeding

Acute gastrointestinal bleeding is a medical emergency. Endoscopy provides therapeutic as well as diagnostic opportunity

The source of obscure gastrointestinal bleeding may be elucidated by angiography, or by isotope scanning techniques

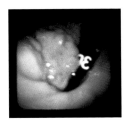 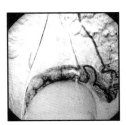 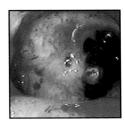 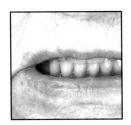

Introduction

Loss of blood from the gastrointestinal tract can be classified according to the site and type of haemorrhage, and the rate of bleeding. Gastrointestinal bleeding occurs predominantly from the upper tract (oesophagus, stomach or duodenum), and also the lower tract (small intestine or colon). Bleeding can be acute or chronic. Chronic bleeding can be apparent or inapparent; in the latter case, bleeding presentation is with anaemia of the iron-deficiency type.

Symptoms
Acute upper gastrointestinal bleeding Haematemesis (vomiting of bright red blood) or 'coffee grounds' (blood denatured by gastric acid), melaena (dark tarry stools) or a combination. Oesophageal bleeding may be frank red, while gastric and duodenal bleeding tend to present with coffee grounds. Gastric, and in particular duodenal, bleeding may present with melaena only.

Acute lower gastrointestinal bleeding Bleeding from haemorrhoids and the left side of the colon may be bright red and/or only slightly dark. Bleeding from the right side of the colon or distal terminal ileum tends to be maroon in colour. Bleeding from colitis is mixed with stool, but blood from vascular anomalies, Meckel's diverticulum, or diverticulae is often separate.

Management and diagnosis
Management and diagnosis of acute bleeding are interrelated.
- Assess severity of blood loss. Transfuse regularly if necessary. Always arrange cross-match.
- Endoscopy (emergency) if bleeding severe or on next available list if less severe.
- Consider therapeutic options (conservative/ transfuse, interventional endoscopy, e.g. sclerotherapy, use of drugs, surgery).
- If emergency endoscopy does not diagnose source/cause of bleeding, and bleeding persists, consider alternative diagnostic techniques – red cell scanning (**267**), angiography, laparotomy.

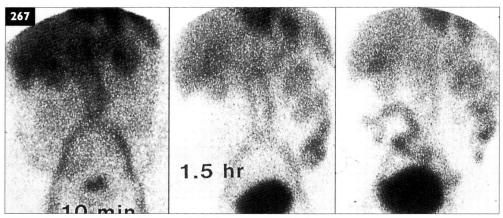

267 Red cell scan, showing (10 minute) labelled red cells in bladder, vascular tree, kidneys, liver and spleen. Over the next 2 hours there is progressive accumulation, commencing in the small bowel on the left side (jejunum).

Acute Upper Gastrointestinal Bleeding

Typical cause include:
- Mallory–Weiss tear.
- Oesophageal varices.
- Oesophagitis.
- Gastric erosions.
- Gastric ulcer.
- Gastric cancer.
- Duodenal ulcer.
- Duodenal erosions.
- Miscellaneous.

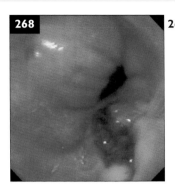

268 Acute Mallory–Weiss tear of the lower oesophagus.

Treatment
Gastrointestinal bleeding may stop spontaneously, but if there is persistent or severe bleeding, active intervention is required to stop bleeding, whether endoscopic, surgical or pharmacological in nature. If urgent intervention not used, later treatment is often necessary to treat underlying disease (e.g. heal duodenal ulceration). If there is persistent acute blood loss (>4 units of blood), particularly in the elderly, the chances that surgery will be needed increase greatly.

MALLORY–WEISS TEAR
This is an acute tear at the oesophagogastric junction which is initiated by retching/vomiting. There is a characteristic history of repeated vomiting – often after alcoholic binging – with vomiting of bright red blood after several episodes of vomiting without blood. Endoscopy shows gaping of mucosa, seen as a linear longitudinal tear at the oesophagogastric junction (**268**).

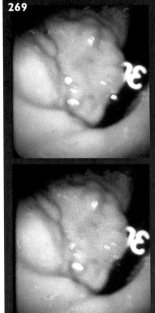

269 Retroflexed view of the fundus of the stomach, showing gastric varices.

Treatment
The condition generally settles spontaneously.

Prognosis
Complete healing is anticipated.

OESOPHAGEAL VARICES
These comprise veins carrying blood from the high-pressure portal system to the systemic circulation, via the lower oesophagus. The condition is generally associated with cirrhosis, and is the most dangerous form of upper gastrointestinal bleeding as it is often associated with liver failure, including coagulopathy.

Endoscopically, the condition appears as dilated varicose vessels in the lower third of the oesophagus; occasionally. there are associated similar varices in the stomach (**269**) or a general congestion of the stomach (portal gastropathy) (**270**).

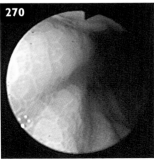

270 The 'snake skin' appearance of portal gastropathy.

Acute Upper Gastrointestinal Bleeding

Diagnostically, the condition can be defined on ultrasound, CT or angiography, but endoscopy is required to confirm whether the varices are bleeding.

Treatment
Active intervention varies:
- Injection sclerotherapy – injecting sclerosant fluid into or adjacent to varices.
- Banding – placing rubber bands, via the endoscope, onto the surface of the varices to obliterate them.
- Balloon tamponade – passage of multibore tubes with two inflatable balloons (Sengstaken– Blakemore tube) which, when inflated, press against bleeding varices to stop bleeding.
- Pharmacological intervention. Intravenous vasopressin or somatostatin reduce portal pressure and aid cessation of haemorrhage. Vasopressin causes systemic vasoconstriction (danger of coronary vasospasm) so simultaneous nitrates are helpful.
- Formation of a portal systemic shunt to decrease portal pressure. This is done either surgically (e.g. portal vein to inferior vena cava); or by interventional radiology – passing a stent from the hepatic vein through the substance of the liver to the portal vein (TIPSS, Transvenous Intrahepatic Portal Systemic Shunt).
- A direct surgical approach to oversew the varices, or to disconnect bleeding varices from the portal circulation by oesophageal transection and reanastomosis.

All such approaches have disadvantages. Sclerotherapy and banding are difficult during severe blood loss. Pharmacological treatment is often ineffective. Balloon tamponade may precipitate ulceration and aspiration pneumonia. The portal systemic shunt precipitates hepatic encephalopathy. Major surgery may be poorly tolerated.

ULCER BLEEDING
This occurs predominantly from duodenal ulcer or gastric ulcers. Both are diagnosed at endoscopy.

Treatment
Acute treatment with local therapy to bleeding gastric and duodenal ulcer is by injection of diluted adrenaline, alcohol, sclerosing fluids, or by use of a heat probe or laser. Such treatment is generally reserved for actively bleeding ulcers, or those with stigmata of recent bleeds (**271, 272**).

Follow-up treatment
Treatment to heal ulcers should be started as soon as practicable, but does not alter the outcome of acute bleeding.

GASTRIC EROSIONS
Diffuse loss of the mucosal epithelium and small ulcers can cause persistent haemorrhage (**273**). This condition is often associated with the use of non-steroidal anti-inflammatory drugs and intake of alcohol. The condition is diagnosed at endoscopy, but treatment may be difficult. Conservative treatment includes a pharmacological approach to reduce splanchnic blood flow (e.g. somatostatin), multiple heat probing or surgery.

MISCELLANEOUS
Small telangiectasia in the stomach or small intestine may bleed (**274, 275**). These may be part of the autosomal dominant familial condition of hereditary haemorrhagic telangiectasia, in which case there may be similar lesions on the face (**276**). Occasionally, large congenital vascular abnormalities involve the small intestine (**277**).

Acute Upper Gastrointestinal Bleeding

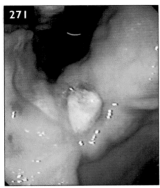

271 Incisural gastric ulcer with evidence of recent bleeding.

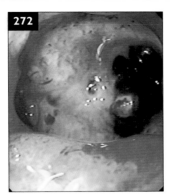

272 Duodenal ulcer with visible vessel in base.

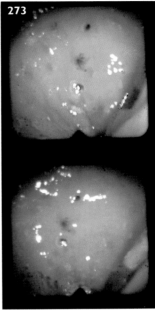

273 Endoscopy of the stomach showing necrotic bleeding antral erosions.

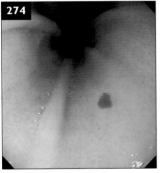

274 Telangiectasia in the stomach.

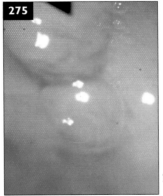

275 Telangiectasia of the ampulla of Vater.

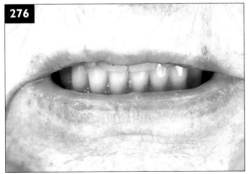

276 Small red telangiectasias seen around the lip (note upper lip) characteristic of Osler Rendu Weber, hereditary haemorrhagic telangiectasia.

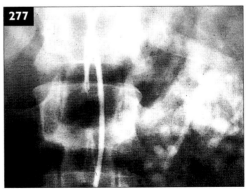

277 A diffuse abnormality affecting the whole of the jejunum (predominantly dilated veins), seen on angiogram.

Lower Gastrointestinal Bleeding

DIVERTICULAR DISEASE
Rarely there may be rapid loss of frank blood from dilated veins in sigmoid colonic diverticula – often 500 ml or more (**278**). Acute diagnosis is by urgent colonoscopy, and is often difficult in the unprepared colon, so diagnosis may be presumptive when subsequent colonoscopy/barium enema shows diverticula. Surgery is rarely indicated. Follow-up treatment is generally conservative; a high-roughage diet may be indicated for diverticulosis.

RECTAL/COLONIC POLYPS
This is seen as intermediate loss of small volumes of blood – often occult – and frequently presents as iron-deficiency anaemia. Diagnosis is by colonoscopy/barium enema in a prepared colon. Colonoscopy offers the opportunity for polypectomy (and therefore also cancer prevention by removal of pre-neoplastic lesions).

ANGIODYSPLASIA
This is an abnormal vasculature developing in the right side of the colon; it is predominantly caecal with advancing age. There are dilated ectatic submucosal blood vessels with both arterial and venous ectasia. The condition presents with intermittent blood loss – either visible (often dark red) – or with iron-deficiency anaemia. For acute diagnosis, the condition may be invisible on barium enema, but may be diagnosed by colonoscopy (with difficulty in an unprepared colon) or by angiography.

For treatment, use colonoscopic diathermy for electrocoagulation of lesions, or resection of affected area.

Haemangiomas are more extensive abnormalities that can present in a similar way (**279, 280**).

COLONIC CANCER
If bleeding, this condition presents with symptoms similar to those of rectal polyp. Severe bleeding occurs only rarely. Right-sided lesions classically present with iron-deficiency anaemia. Diagnosis is by colonoscopy or barium enema. Treatment is with surgical resection.

ISCHAEMIC COLITIS
Symptoms include dark red bleeding, mixed with the stools in elderly patients, and often associated with pain. The condition affects the splenic flexure, descending colon (the most vulnerable area of the colon 'watershed' area between inferior and superior mesenteric artery territories). Diagnosis is by plain abdominal radiograph, which may show 'thumb-printing' of ischaemic colon in the splenic flexure. Treatment is conservative as the colitis generally stops. Later consequences may include stricture which occasionally requires resection.

OTHER CAUSES
Ulcerative colitis or bacillary dysentery both cause rectal bleeding, but this is part of an exudative diarrhoea, with pus, mucus and tenesmus. Haemorrhoidal bleeding has the characteristics of oozing post-defaecation (bright red blood), often after passage of hard stools. Blood is only often noticed on the toilet paper or in the lavatory pan. Such blood loss is only very rarely sufficient to cause anaemia.

GASTROINTESTINAL BLEEDING: SOME GENERAL POINTS
In obscure/recurrent gastrointestinal bleeding – that which has been undiagnosed after routine endoscopy and radiograph of the upper and lower gastrointestinal tract – consider:
• Visceral angiography.
• Exploratory laparotomy.

Angiography may either show an abnormality, which can potentially bleed (e.g. angiodysplasia of the caecum), or in acute cases blood loss can be demonstrated actrively by leakages of contrast medium into the bowel lumen. Therefore the procedure can be used in both acute and chronic bleeding

In young patients, most causes of obscure gastrointestinal bleeding would be readily found by the surgeon at laparotomy (e.g. Meckel's diverticulum or tumours). In elderly patients, vascular anomalies are the dominant cause of bleeding, and routine laparotomy does not demonstrate this. Specialised techniques such as on-table total endoscopy with trans-illumination of the bowel may help to show vascular anomalies at surgery.

Lower Gastrointestinal Bleeding

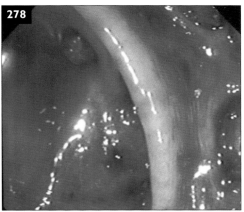

278 Diverticulosis, seen in the setting of a recent rectal bleed.

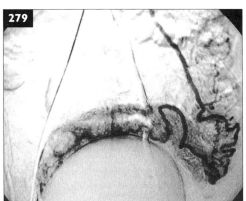

279 Inferior mesenteric artery angiogram showing gross arterial and venous anomalies in the sigmoid colon (haemangioma).

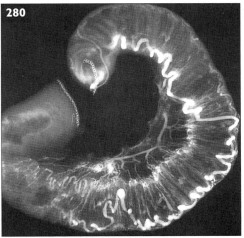

280 Resected specimen from the previous angiogram (**279**); the same vascular pattern, here injected with barium, is clearly seen.

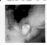

Small-Intestinal Bleeding

MECKEL'S DIVERTICULUM

This is a remnant of the embryonic vitellointestinal duct, situated 60 cm from the ileocaecal valve (**281**). It is the cause of intermittent blood loss which is seen as a deep maroon-coloured stool, and may be associated with a history of postprandial pain. The condition is caused by ulceration of the ectopic gastric mucosa in the diverticulum. Meckel's scan (⁹⁹ᵐTechnetium scanning) (**282**) may show excretion of the isotope by the ectopic gastric mucosa, but is not reliable.

Other causes

Other causes of small-intestinal bleeding have been identified. Although rare, these include:
- Ulcers induced by non-steroidal anti-inflammatory drugs.
- Tumours – carcinoma, lymphoma, leiomyoma (tumour of smooth muscle).

- Vascular anomalies (haemangioma, angiodysplasia). Blood loss may be obvious (generally melaena-like) or inapparent (in which case presentation is with iron-deficiency anaemia).

Diagnosis

This is often difficult because:
- Small-intestinal causes of blood loss are often not considered.
- Such problems are generally beyond reach of routine endoscopy. Enteroscopy can now visualise the small intestine, but enteroscopes differ, either visualising only the upper portion of the jejunum or, in a prolonged procedure, more of the small intestine to the ileum. However, this technique is not widely used.
- Barium studies of the small intestine are difficult to interpret. However, angiography may be helpful (**277**).

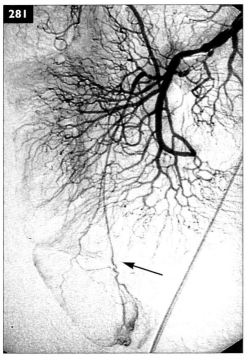

281 Angiogram outlining a Meckel's diverticulum, fed by a long aberrant vessel (arrowed).

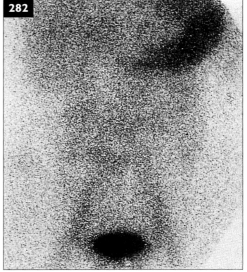

282 A Meckel's scan. There is normal excretion of ⁹⁹ᵐpertechnetate shown in the bladder and in the stomach, and a dubious area of accumulation in the right iliac fossa (just seen to the right of the V shown by the iliac vessels). Generally, this is not a good test and both false negatives and dubious false positives are common.

Chapter Ten

Miscellaneous Conditions

Constipation may reflect lifestyle or disease

Ascites may reflect hepatic, cardiac, renal, intestinal or primary peritoneal disease

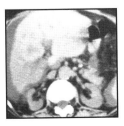 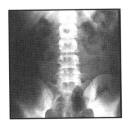 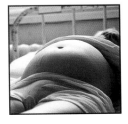 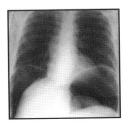

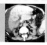

Ascites

Definition
Ascites is defined as the accumulation of fluid in peritoneal cavity (**283–285**). Such accumulation occurs due to one or more of:
- Local exudation from the peritoneum.
- Hypoproteinaemia.
- High pressure in the portal or systemic venous systems.

Causes
The causes of ascites may reflect local or general problems.

General problems:
- Cardiac failure/constrictive pericarditis (associated with peripheral oedema and elevated jugular venous pressure).
- Renal failure (associated with marked urinary protein loss).
- Liver failure.
- Low protein states, e.g. kwashiorkor (protein malnutrition) or protein-losing enteropathy.

Local problems:
- Peritoneal exudation, e.g. tuberculous peritonitis.
- Peritoneal malignancy: primary – mesothelioma (suspect also asbestos exposure); secondary adenocarcinoma (ovarian common, or colon, stomach or pancreas).

Investigations
- Exclude renal and cardiac causes by examination of jugular venous pressure and urine. Exclude gynaecological malignancy (pelvic examination).
- Examine for stigmata of chronic liver disease.
- Ultrasound – for evidence of chronic liver disease (abnormal liver, splenomegaly, abnormal collaterals). Ultrasound is the most sensitive means of detecting small volumes of ascites, as well as for pelvic and other malignancy.
- Paracentesis – examine for appearances (blood suggests malignancy), protein concentration. Former distinction into transudate (<20 g/l protein) and exudate (>30 g/l) used to suggest cirrhosis (low protein) or infection (high protein) has been replaced by consideration of the albumin serum–ascites gradient. (see *Table* 5). Cytology and culture (>250 × 10⁶/l, cf normal peripheral blood count 4,000–9,000 × 10⁶/l neutrophil, leucocytes) suggests

infection; this is particularly likely to occur when ascites is a complication of hepatic disease).
- CT demonstrates liver outline and liver tumours, alterations in mesentery and peritoneum, and pelvic malignancy (though can be false positive in this area).
- Laparoscopy/peritoneal biopsy.

Management
Reverse precipitating causes if possible. In liver disease (cirrhosis), diuretics should be used judiciously, as only 750 ml of ascitic fluid can be reabsorbed spontaneously from the peritoneal cavity, so a steady weight loss of >0.75 kg/day, in the absence of peripheral oedema, may initiate hypovolaemia. Recently, large-volume paracentesis (6 l/day) with replacement of albumin (6–8 g/l of ascites), has been introduced for rapid mobilisation of ascites in liver disease.

Ascites

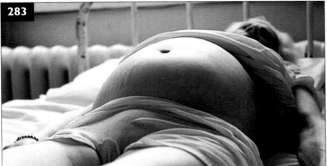

283 Ascites.

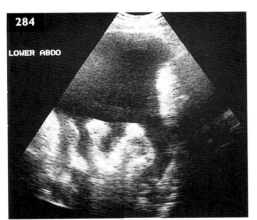

284 Ascites. The ultrasound shows the appearance of loops of bowel floating in echo-free ascitic fluid.

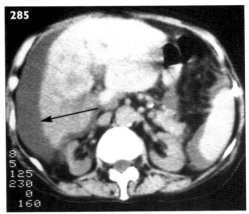

285 CT scan. The area of ascites is best seen as the light grey area lateral to the liver (arrow).

Table 5. Causes of ascites – graduated according to whether the gradient of albumin concentration between serum and ascites is high or low

High gradient ascites Gradient >11 g/l	Low gradient ascites Gradient <11 g/l
Cirrhosis	Peritoneal carcinomatosis
Alcoholic hepatitis	TB peritonitis
Cardiac ascites	Pancreatic ascites
Massive metastases	Biliary ascites
Fulminant hepatic failure	Nephrotic syndrome
Budd-Chiari syndrome	Serositis
Veno-occlusive disease	
Fatty liver	
Myxoedema	

Constipation

Definition
First of all, it is important to find out what the patient means!

Absolute constipation is defined as the failure to pass any stool. If this is associated with pain and distension, then obstruction must be suspected. Otherwise, constipation generally means infrequent passage of stools (normal frequency varies between three times daily to every 3 days) or passage of very hard stools, even with normal frequency (**286**). In the elderly, severe constipation and straining may be associated with rectal prolapse.

The causes of constipation include:
- Inadequate food intake.
- Lack of exercise (profound immobility, e.g. multiple sclerosis, age).
- Lack of roughage (undigested vegetable matter).
- Obstructive lesions in the lumen (e.g. colonic cancer)
- Diverticular disease (narrow sigmoid due to muscle hypertrophy).
- Hirschsprung's disease.

Treatment
- Initially, organic causes should be excluded – use a barium enema. This is not always needed, and particularly not in young patients with a long-standing history of non-progressive disease.
- Increase exercise in idiopathic types.
- Use of laxatives. Osmotic laxatives (lactulose, magnesium salts) are much preferable to stimulant laxatives (e.g. senna), as prolonged use of stimulant laxatives leads to the destruction of nerve ganglia.

INCONTINENCE
Faecal incontinence is defined as the involuntary passage of faecal matter and has a variety of causes:
- Acute diarrhoeal states. e.g. gastroenteritis.
- Colonic motility abnormalities, e.g. extreme fright. Incontinence occurs only rarely in irritable bowel or in hormone-mediated diarrhoea.
- Anal sphincter dysfunction. This occurs mainly in elderly patients, but also occasionally with severe perianal Crohn's disease, or after injudicious surgery for perianal fistulae.
- Neurological problems – pressure on the spinal cord. (this is generally associated with urinary sphincter abnormality).

In the elderly, severe constipation can lead to 'overflow incontinence' with the passage of liquid stools forced past obvious hard faeces in the rectum.

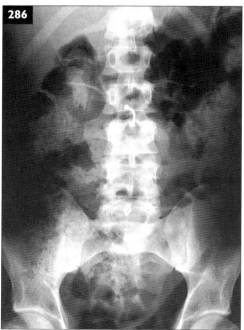

286 Plain abdominal X-ray showing mottled accumulation of faecal matter in ascending colon.

Acute Peritonitis

Definition
Inflammation of peritoneum, associated with pain and tenderness when the parietal peritoneum is inflamed. The condition gives local signs, e.g. tenderness over inflamed appendix. A perforated gut generally leads to generalised peritonitis (classically perforated duodenal ulcer) and causes board-like rigidity of abdomen. Perforation may however be localised (e.g. from colonic diverticula), giving only localised tenderness.

Investigations
Typically, the white cell count will be elevated. A plain radiograph may show free air if the peritonitis precipitated by perforation (287). Serum amylase levels will be markedly increased in acute pancreatitis which, when very severe, can give rise to generalised peritonitis. However, perforation of the upper gastrointestinal tract can moderately elevate serum amylase (loss of amylase-rich fluid from the duodenum into the peritoneum and hence into the circulation).

Management
Rapid resuscitation is important (marked loss of fluid and protein into the peritoneal cavity will induce hypovolaemia). Generally urgent surgical intervention. Antibiotic therapy should be for wide coverage, including Gram-negative anaerobes.

SPONTANEOUS BACTERIAL PERITONITIS
This is a complication of pre-existing ascites, particularly in cirrhotic patients, and is due to the passage of bacteria through the gut wall in the absence of frank perforation. The condition should be considered if a patient with cirrhosis and ascites deteriorates non-specifically. Investigation is by paracentesis. There is an elevated white cell count ($>250 \times 10^6/l$ polymorphonuclear leucocytes). Treatment is with broad-spectrum antibiotics.

TUBERCULOUS PERITONITIS
This condition presents with a doughy abdomen, and high-protein ascites with lymphocyte predominance. Acid-fast bacilli are often not cultured. Laparoscopy may help in the diagnosis, or a therapeutic trial of anti-tuberculosis treatment.

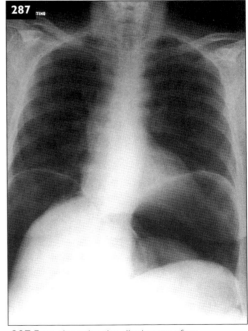

287 Free air under the diaphragm after perforation of the gut.

Appendix

Causes of abdominal pain

Causes of dysphagia

Major GI causes of anaemia

Causes of acute GI bleeding

Causes of protein-losing enteropathy

Causes of abnormal small intestine biopsies with villous abnormalities causing malabsorption in adults

Causes of constipation

Screening blood tests for GI disease

Causes of diarrhoea and malabsorption

Anatomical investigations and potential value in chronic diarrhoea and malabsorption

Normal ranges urine: values per 24-hour excretion

Normal ranges faeces: values per 24-hour excretion

Normal ranges, plasma/serum

Gastric function tests – gastric acid secretion mmols per hour

Tests for malabsorption

Appendix

Table 6. Causes Of Abdominal Pain

Gastro-duodenal disorders
Non-ulcer dyspepsia
Peptic ulcer
Acute gastritis
Tumours

Biliary disorders
Gallstones
Acute cholecystitis
Biliary colic

Hepatic causes
Hepatic congestion
(cardiac failure, hepatic
venous congestion)
Acute hepatitis
Hepatic tumours

Pancreatic causes
Acute pancreatitis
Chronic pancreatitis
Pancreatic carcinoma
Pseudocysts
Abscesses

Small intestinal disorders
Motility disorders - irritable bowel
Ischaemic gut
Inflammatory bowel disease
Obstruction
Pseudo-obstruction

Colonic disorders
Motility disorders- irritable bowel,
cathartic colon,
Diverticulitis
Obstruction
Pericolic abscess
Ischaemic bowel

Miscellaneous
Lead poisoning
Tabes dorsalis
Central
Porphyria

Table 7. Causes Of Dysphagia

Central
Bulbar palsy
Psedobulbar palsy
Globus hystericus

Local Oral
Ulcerative stomatitis
Painful glossitis
Dental problems

Pharyngeal
Muscular weakness/incoordination
Pharyngeal pouch
Extrinsic compression (tumours, lym-
phadenopathy, etc)

Oesophageal
Muscular incoordination
  Achalasia
  Spasm
  Systemic sclerosis
  Presby-oesophagus
Webs
Benign strictures
Malignant strictures
Extrinsic compression

Appendix

Table 8. Major GI Causes Of Anaemia

Iron deficiency
Chronic bleeding – NSAIDs treatment, peptic ulcer,
Oesphagitis, IBD, adenomas, carcinomas)
Malabsorptive states
Post-gastrectomy
Dietary inadequacy

Folate deficiency
Malabsorptive states
Inflammatory bowel disease
Dietary inadequacy

B$_{12}$ deficiency
Atrophic gastritis (pernicious anaemia)
Postgastrectomy
Ileal disease and resection
Bacterial overgrowth
Pancreatic disease
Strict vegetarianism

Anaemia of chronic disease
Inflammatory bowel disease
Disseminated malignancy

Acute blood loss
GI bleeding

Table 9. Causes Of Acute GI Bleeding

Upper GI Causes
Common
Gastric and duodenal erosions
Peptic ulcer
Mallory-Weiss tear
Oesophageal varices

Less common
Oesophageal ulcers/oesophagitis
Gastric tumours
Vascular anomalies

Lower GI Causes
Haemorrhoids
Diverticular bleeding
Inflammatory bowel disease
Adenomas
Carcinomas
Ischaemic colitis
Angiodysplasia
Meckel's diverticulum
Intussusception

Less common (both upper and lower)
Vasculitis
Bleeding disorders
Small bowel tumours
Small bowel angiomas
Pseudoxanthoma elasticum
Ehlers Danlos syndrome

Appendix

Table 10. Causes Of Protein-Losing Enteropathy

Primary lymphangiectasia
Secondary lymphangiectasia
Giant rugal hypertrophy of stomach
(Ménétrier's)
Zollinger Ellison
Inflammatory bowel disease
Carcinomas
Constricitive pericarditis
Whipple's disease
Coeliac disease

Table 11. Causes of Abnormal Small Intestine Biopsies with Villous Abnormalities Causing Malabsorption in Adults

Coeliac disease
Dermatitis herpetiformis
Ulcerative ileojejunitis
Whipple's disease
Immunodeficiency
Lymphoma
Crohn's disease
Severe radiation enteritis
Graft versus host disease

Table 12. Causes of Constipation

Inadequate dietary Intake
Inadequate roughage (dietary fibre)
Immobility
Obstructing lesions in bowel
Ileus and Pseudo-obstruction
Purgative abuse (cathartic colon)
Pregnancy
Depression
Drugs (opiates, anticholinergics,
beta-blockers, calcium and
aluminium-containing antacids, etc)
Paraplegia
Hirschprung's disease
Metabolic causes (myxoedema, low
potassium, hypercalcaemia)

Table 13. Screening Blood Tests for GI Disease

Full blood count
Biochemical profile
ESR
C-reactive protein
Serum iron and iron binding capacity
Serum folate and B_{12}
Suspected malabsorption – add
    Immunoglobulins
    Endomysial antibody
Consider HIV testing

Appendix

Table 14. Causes Of Diarrhoea And Malabsorption

Gastric causes
Post-gastrectomy
Gastrinoma – Zollinger-Ellison
Post-vagotomy
Achlorhydria, predisposing to bacterial overgrowth
Gastro-enteric fistulae and gastro-enterostomy

Pancreatic causes
Chronic pancreatitis
Pancreatic resection
Carcinoma
Cystic fibrosis
Schwachman's syndrome
Congenital enzyme deficien

Hepatobiliary causes
Cholestasis
Bile-salt therapy

Small intestinal causes
Short gut syndrome
Ileal resection
Lactase deficiency
Coeliac disease
Dermatitis herpetiformis
Ulcerative ileo-jejunitis
Tropical sprue
Post-infectious malabsorption
Whipple's disease
Lymphangiectasia
Lymphoma
Bacterial overgrowth
Infections - viral, bacterial, protozoal
Immunodeficiency including AIDS
Radiation enteritis
Food allergies
Eosinophilic enteritis
Mesenteric ischaemia

Vasculitis
Abetalipoproteinaemia
Amyloidosis
Autonomic neuropathy
Visceral myopathy
Graft versus host disease
Systemic sclerosis
Entero-colic fistula

Colonic causes
Colonic resection
Infections
Ulcerative colitis
Crohn's disease
Irritable bowel
Diverticular disease
Pseudomembranous colitis
Constipation with overflow
Microscopic colitis
Collagenous colitis
Radiation colitis
Purgative abuse (cathartic colon)
Villous adenoma
Carcinoma
Graft versus host disease

Endocrine causes
Diabetes
Carcinoid syndrome
VIPOMA
Thyrotoxicosis
Addison's disease
Zollinger-Ellison
Medullary carcinoma of thyroid

Drugs
Very many – magnesium-containing antacids, antibiotics, purgatives, cytotoxics, etc.

Appendix

Table 15. Anatomical Investigations and Potential Value in Chronic Diarrhoea and Malabsorption

Endoscopic duodenal/jejunal biopsy
Coeliac disease
Tropical sprue
Lymphoma
Whipple's disease
Alpha-chain disease
Giardiasis
HIV enteropathy
Mycobacterium avium intracellulare
Lymphangiectasia
Kaposi's

Small intestinal radiology
Malabsorptive pattern
Crohn's disease
Jejunal diverticulosis
Lymphangiectasia
Lymphoma
Blind-loops
Resection
Entero-enteric connections
Pseudo-obstruction
Strictures
TB
Whipple's disease
Nodular lymphoid hyperplasia

Sigmoidoscopy, colonoscopy and biopsy
Ulcerative colitis
Crohn's disease
Diverticulitis
Minimal change and collagenous colitis
Melanosis coli
Amoebiasis
Amyloidosis
Lymphoma
Carcinoma

Barium enema
Carcinoma
Ulcerative colitis
Crohn's disease
Diverticular disease
Ischaemic colitis
Cathartic colon
Fistula
TB

ERCP
Chronic pancreatitis
Cancer of pancreas
Cholestatic liver disease

Appendix

NORMAL RANGES

Note: All normal ranges should be checked against local laboratory reference ranges. This applies to all tests, but in particular should be noted with dynamic tests (e.g., acid secretion) and immunoassays.

Table 16. Normal Ranges Urine: Values per 24-hour Excretion

Constituent	SI or other International units	Traditional units
Amino acid nitrogen-free	4–20 mmol	50–300 mg
Amylase	200–1500 U	10–7000 Henry–Chiamori units
Calcium	2.5–7.5 mmol	100–300 mg
Copper	0.2–1.5 µmol	10–100 µg
Creatinine	9–18 mmol	1.0–2.0 g
Glucose	0.1–1.0 mmol	20–200 mg
5-Hydroxy-indoleacetic acid	10–45 µmol	2–8 mg
Indicans	0.1–0.4 mmol	20–80 mg
Lead	0–0.3 µmol	0–60 µg
Nitrogen – total	0.7–1.5 mol	10–20 g
Osmolality	700–1500 mmol	700–1500 mosmol
Phosphate	15–50 mmol	0.5–1.5 g
Porphyrins		
δ-Aminolaevulinic acid	1–40 µmol	0.1–5.0 mg
Porphobilinogen	1–12 µmol	0.2–2.0 mg
Coproporphyrin	0.15–0.3 µmol	100–200 µg
Uroporphyrin	6–40 nmol	5–30 µg
Potassium	40–120 mmol	40–120 mEq
Protein – total	40–120 mg	40–120 mg
Sodium	100–250 mmol	100–250 mEq

Table 17. Normal Ranges Faeces: Values per 24-hour Excretion

Constituent	SI or other international units	Traditional units
Total wet weight	60–250 g	60–250 g
Total dry weight	20–60 g	20–60 g
Fat – total	10–18 mmol	3–5 g
Nitrogen – total	70–110 mmol	1–1.5 g

Appendix

Table 18. Normal Ranges, Plasma/Serum

Constituent	SI or other international units	Traditional units
Amino acid nitrogen	2.5–4.0 mmol/l	3.5–5.5 mg/100 ml
Ammonia (whole blood)	12–60 µmol/l	20–100 µg/100 ml
Amylase	70–300 U/l	40–160 Somogyi units/100 ml
Anion gap	6–16 mmol/l	6–16 mEq/l
Bicarbonate	24–30 mmol/l	24–30 mEq/l
Bilirubin		
total	5.0–17 µmol/l	0.3–1.0 mg/100 ml
conjugated	<3.0 µmol/l	<0.2 mg/100 ml
Caeruloplasmin	0.3–0.6 g/l	30–60 mg/100 ml
Calcium	2.1–2.6 mmol/l	8.5–10.5 mg/l00 ml
Carbon dioxide (whole blood)	4.5–6.0 kPa	35–46 mmHg
Carbonic acid	1.1–1.4 mmol/l	1.1–1.4 mEq/l
Carotenoids	1.0–5.5 µmol/l	50–300 µg/100 ml
Chloride	95–105 mmol/l	95–105 mEq/l
Cholesterol – total	4.0–6.5 mmol/l	160–260 mg/100 ml
Copper	13–24 µmol/l	80–150 µg/100 ml
Cortisol	200–700 nmol/l	8–35 µg/100 ml
Creatinine	60–120 µmol/l	0.7–1.4 mg/100 ml
Creatine kinase	3–150 U/l	3–150 iu/l
Fatty acids – free	0.3–0.6 mmol/l	0.3–0.6 mEq/l
Ferritin	15–250 µg/l	1.5–25 µg/100 ml
Folate	5.0–20 µg/l	5.0–20 ng/ml
Gastrin	5–50 pmol/l	10–100 pg/ml
Glucose (whole blood)		
venous	3.0–5.0 mmol/l	55–90 mg/100 ml
capillary	3.2–5.2 mmol/l	60–95 mg/100 ml
γ-Glutamyltransferase	5–45 U/l	5–45 iu/l
Haptoglobins	5–30 µmol/l	30–180 mg/100 ml
Iron	11–34 µmol/l	60–190 µg/100 ml
Iron-binding capacity – total	45–75 µmol/l	250–400 µg/100 ml
Ketones	0.06–0.2 mmol/l	0.06–0.2 mEq/l
Lactate	0.75–2.0 mmol/l	0.75–2.0 mEq/l
Lead (whole blood)	0.5–1.7 µmol/l	10–35 µg/100 ml

Appendix

Table 18. Normal Ranges, Plasma/Serum contd.

Constituent	SI or other international units	Traditional units
Lipase	18–280 U/l	0–1.5 Cherry–Crandall units
Lipids – total fasting	4.5–10 g/l	450–1000 mg/100 ml
Magnesium	0.7–1.0 mmol/l	1.8–2.4 mg/100 ml
5'-Nucleotidase	2–15 U/l	2–15 iu/l
Osmolality	275–295 mmol/kg	275–295 mosmol/kg
Oxygen (whole blood)	11–15 kPa	85–105 mmHg
pH	7.36–7.42	7.36–7.42
Phosphatases		
acid – total	0.5–5.5 U/l	0.3–3.0 KAu/100 ml
– 'prostatic'	0–1 U/l	0–0.5 KAu/100 ml
alkaline – total	20–95 U/l	3–13 KAu/100 ml
Phosphate – inorganic	0.8–1.4 mmol/l	2.5–4.5 mg/100 ml
Phospholipids	1.8–3.0 mmol/l	150–250 mg/100 ml
Potassium	3.5–5.0 mmol/l	3.5–5.0 mEq/l
Protein		
Total	60–80 g/l	6.0–8.0 g/100 ml
Albumin	35–50 g/l	3.5–5.0 g/100 ml
Globulin – total	18–32 g/l	1.8–3.2 g/100 ml
γ-Globulin – total	7–15 g/l	0.7–1.5 g 100 ml
IgA	1.0–4.0 g/l	100–400 mg/100 ml
IgG	8.0–16.0 g/l	800–1600 mg/100 ml
IgM	0.5–2.5 g/l	50–250 mg/100 ml
Fibrinogen	2–4 g/l	0.2–0.4 g/100 ml
Sodium	135–145 mmol/l	135–145 mEq/l
Transaminases		
alanine	5–25 U/l	5–25 iu/l
aspartate	5–35 U/l	5–35 iu/l
Transferrin	1.2–2.0 g/l	120–200 mg/100 ml
Triglyceride	0.3–1.8 mmol/l	25–150 mg/100 ml
Trypsin	140–400 µg/l	140–400 ng/ml
Urea	3.0–6.5 mmol/l	18–40 mg/100 ml
Urate	0.1–0.4 mmol/l	1.5–7.0 mg/100 ml
VIP	<5 pmol/l	
Vitamin A	1.0–3.0 µmol/l	30–90 µg/100 ml
Vitamin B12	160–900 ng/l	160–900 pg/ml
Vitamin D	8–60 nmol/l	3–4 ng/ml
Zinc	12–17 µmol/l	80–110 µg/100 ml

Appendix

DYNAMIC TESTS

Table 19. Gastric Function Tests – Gastric Acid Secretion mmols per Hour

Ulcer	Normal		Duodenal	
	Basal	Peak	Basal	Peak
Men	1 (0-5)	22 (1-45)	4 (0-15)	42 (15-100)
Women	1 (0-5)	12 (1–30)	2 (0–5)	32 (15–100)
	Zollinger–Ellison			
	Basal	Peak		
Typical	15–30	60–120		

Note: The significant difference noted in Zollinger–Ellison is the high basal as well as the high peak acid ouput. In addition ZE has high-fasting gastrin (>60 pg/ml) – should be tested off acid suppressant drugs for adequate time (days to weeks) as achlorhydria also gives high gastrin levels.

Table 20. Tests for Malabsorption

Fat
3-day faecal fat >18 mmol or 6 g fat per day when on 70 g fat intake.

Carbohydrate – Xylose tolerance test
Typically 25 g oral xylose. >25% ingested dose after 6 hours in urine (Note: this requires normal renal function). 1- or 2-hour blood estimations may be performed.

Lactose tolerance test
This tests for disaccharidase deficiency and should normally show a rise in blood glucose of 20 mg/dl after 50 g lactose. Clinically, whether this provokes symptoms of diarrhoea and flatulence is also helpful.

Pancreatic function testing
1. PABA test. >50% ingested PABA (500–1.5 g orally) in urine over 6 hours. (Note: this requires normal renal function).
2. Pancreolauryl secretion. >30% ingested dose in urine over 6 hours.

Index

Index

Index

Index